PHONOLOGY INTRODUCED

Linguistic Development, Speech Pathology, and Communicative Disorders

First Edition

Kimberly Frazier
University of Arkansas - Fayetteville

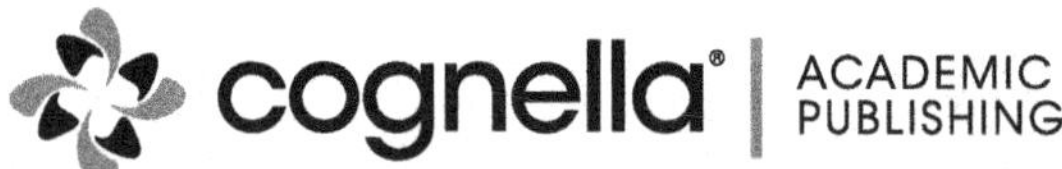

Bassim Hamadeh, CEO and Publisher

Kassie Graves, Director of Acquisitions and Sales

Jamie Giganti, Senior Managing Editor

Miguel Macias, Senior Graphic Designer

Angela Schultz, Acquisitions Editor

Michelle Piehl, Project Editor

Trey Soto, Licensing Coordinator

Berenice Quirino, Associate Production Editor

Bryan Mok, Interior Designer

Printed in the United States of America

ISBN: 978-1-63487-810-4 (pbk) / 978-1-63487-811-1 (br) / 978-1-5165-2763-2 (pf)

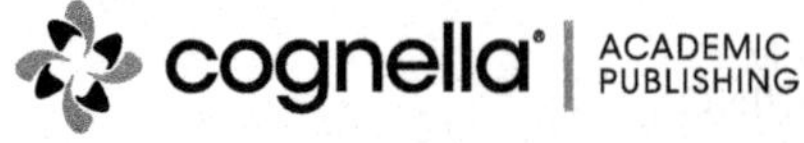

TABLE OF CONTENTS

CHAPTER

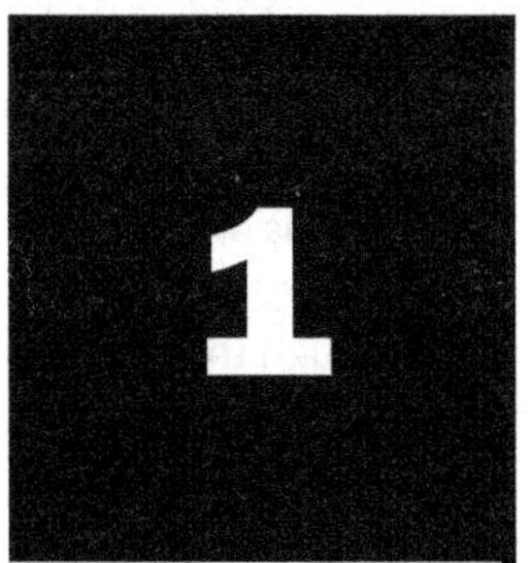

Speech is fleeting—once a word has been uttered, it cannot be unuttered, nor can it be held in memory for analysis unless it is captured in some way. For the speech-language pathologist (SLP), it is necessary to have a visual mechanism for capturing the precise manner in which speech is produced, because it offers the best method for analysis and the appropriate diagnoses of speech disorders and the development of therapeutic interventions. Transcription is the sound-by-sound recording of speech sounds. Knowledge of the International Phonetic Alphabet (IPA) and an understanding of phonology are powerful tools that allow the SLP to visualize speech to diagnose disorders, develop interventions, and also track client progress, because phonetic transcription offers a permanent record of speech.

WHY IPA

The alphabet and orthography (the use of letters to form words) are not sufficient for clinical purposes. To fully understand the magnitude of how orthography falls short, consider the following: There are only 26 letters (graphemes) in the English alphabet representing at least 43 speech sounds, and due to the dynamic nature of language, these 43 speech sounds can be arranged using the alphabet in over 250 ways to spell words (Moats, 1995). For example, the digraph (two letters representing one speech sound) "sh" has more than 20 different spellings. Chandelier, sugar, shoe, fiction, social, mission, ocean, and complexion represent just a few of the common and less common spellings of the "sh" sound. The words *saw* and *was* provide another example—orthographically, the two words appear to be mirror images, and one might assume that they have identical syllable structure and speech sounds. However, this is not at all the case. *Saw* consists of only two speech sounds /sɔ/ while *was* consists of 3 different speech sounds /wʌz/. Singh and Singh (2006) suggested that gaps exist between a language's sound system and written system, because spoken languages evolve while written systems do not change but are instead "ingrained in the orthographic convention" (p. 22).

A BRIEF HISTORY OF OUR MODERN ALPHABET

It is not known how early man's vocal utterances became language expressed through speech that led to the more than 7,000 languages spoken today (Ladefoged, 2005). It is known, however, that one of the greatest feats of mankind was the invention of symbols to stand for speech sounds. These are known as alphabets. At some point, individuals must have come to realize that their language was composed of different speech sounds to have classified the sounds and assigned symbols to them. The modern English alphabet evolved through the efforts of traders, victors of war, missionaries, and scholars over a period of hundreds of years. This cobbled together history, unfortunately, didn't result in the most intuitive and easy-to-use alphabet. The English alphabet and all modern phonetic alphabets have a Phoenician origin (Van Riper & Smith, 1992). Cuneiform and Egyptian hieroglyphic pictographs were the precursors to this alphabet. The inhabitants of Phoenicia were a Semitic people who lived on the coast of the Mediterranean Sea. Phoenicia was so named, because of the coveted purple dye produced from the murex snail native to the region. Because of this prime location, the residents of the area were heavily involved in maritime trading (Mark, 2009) and known throughout as the "traders of purple." This early alphabet is thought to have consisted of symbols representing consonant speech sounds only (McCarter, 1974). Vowels were missing but are crucial in differentiating words. Does one want a pat, pet, pot, pit or putt? It is the vowel that makes the distinction. Around 800 B.C., the Greeks adopted the Semitic alphabet; shortened it somewhat, because their language didn't include certain sounds, such as gutterals; and replaced some of the symbols for consonants with vowels (McCarter, 1974). The alphabet allowed the Greeks to write down their stories and poems. The Romans, known as "Latins" at the time, adapted the Greek alphabet and expanded the number of vowels, but they just didn't take the vowel expansion quite far enough. Instead, they were the ones who came up with the idea of putting two vowel symbols together to form a different vowel sound instead of creating a unique symbol. The Latin alphabet resembles the symbols used today. Although there are some variations among the different languages, over 1,000 different languages use the Roman alphabet presently. As Roman missionaries spread the Christian religion to England and other conquered territories, the Latin alphabet spread as well and was used by the educated elite of the region (McCarter, 1974). The invention of the printing press in 1448 produced a more standardized English alphabet. The result of this history is an inconsistent language of complex rules with many exceptions to those rules and an alphabet that is an inadequate tool for the SLP.

Yes, English can be weird.
It can be understood through tough, thorough thought, though.

INTERNATIONAL PHONETIC ALPHABET

The International Phonetic Association, created in 1888, is a universal alphabet containing unique symbols to represent each speech sound used in languages produced throughout the world. It is also the most utilized alphabet in phonetic transcription (Singh & Singh, 2006). Because IPA is "international," it comprises more symbols than is required to represent American English. This text will be concerned primarily with the 44 phonemes spoken in American English. IPA is based on the Latin alphabet but does contain non-Latin symbols, as well. The symbols are enclosed in either brackets [ ] or virgules / / to denote that they do not represent the spelling system of any specific language. For example, the sound "sh" in the English word "shop" is transcribed as /ʃ/ or [ʃ].

IPA provides the perfect tool for making a permanent visual representation of speech sounds as they are heard, rather than how they are spelled. Approximately 44 of these symbols represent the consonants and vowels used in American English. Roughly 14 vowels, 4 diphthongs, 2 triphthongs, and 24 consonants, depending on regional dialects, make-up the 44 symbols introduced in this text.

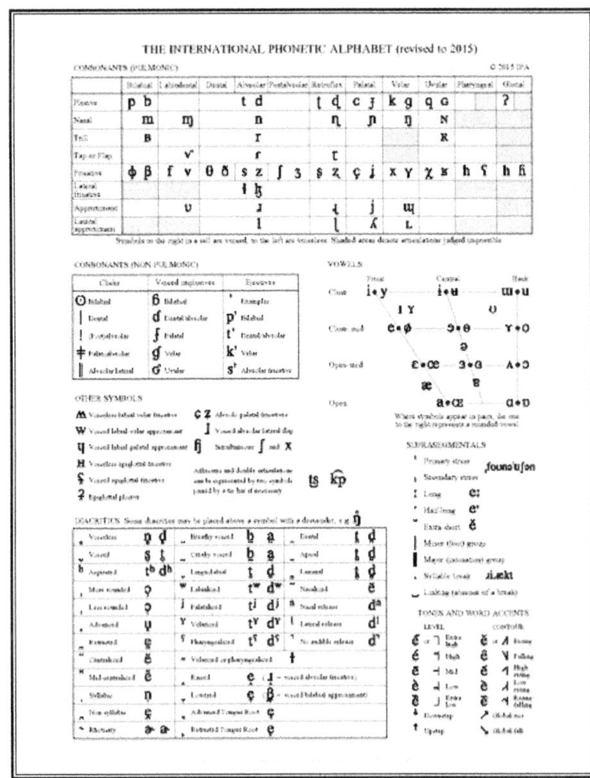

Fig. 1.1: The International Phonetic Alphabet

SPEECH AND LANGUAGE

What is speech? What is language? Speech is a verbal means of expressing information to meet one's needs through a modification of the voiced and unvoiced breath stream through a series of complex motor movements. Language is an agreed upon and socially shared rule-based mechanism to convey information. Language is dynamic, is evolving, and has many forms. It can be spoken or written and even represented through signs or Braille for those with sensory impairments. Speech is not language, but it is the most common mode of expressing language due to its efficiency. Speech is the combination of articulated sounds and prosody. Prosody is a general term referring to the acoustic characteristics of speech for which subtle variations alter the meaning of utterances and give indications about the talker's state of mind. Prosodic features are expressed in spoken language as a suprasegmental "overlay" to the speech sounds being articulated. While prosody does not change the identity of the individual phonemes themselves, it influences the duration, intensity, pitch, and quality of sounds, thereby varying the meaning and emotional content of an utterance (Gerken & McGregor, 1998). Due to technological advances, written language is being used more and more in daily routines, particularly through social media and email. Unfortunately, while this is an effective mechanism in modern society for conveying information to greater numbers of people living near or far, much meaning and intention are lost, because it is impossible to express prosody through written language. In addition to the expression of language and prosody, speech also signals speaker identity. When receiving a phone call, it may be evident from the caller's voice whether it is a dear friend, a family member, a casual acquaintance, or a stranger.

Five rule systems interplay to form language: morphology, phonology, syntax, semantics, and pragmatics. Rules for how sounds form morphemes is known as phonology; rules for how morphemes form words is known as morphology; rules for how words form sentences is known as syntax; rules for how words express meaning is known as semantics; and rules for how these four systems are used in a social context is known as pragmatics. This text will be primarily concerned with the rules of phonology and morphology.

PHONOLOGY AND PHONETICS

Phonology deals with the sound system of a language and the rules for how speech sounds (phonemes) are used to form words. It is vital for SLPs to understand these rules (Van Riper & Smith, 1979). This text will introduce rules of phonology that have specific importance to the SLP.

Phonetics is the study of classifying speech sounds and describing how they are produced (Edwards & Shriberg, 1983). The study of phonetics is devoted to describing and classifying speech sounds as they are actually produced and how they sound to the listener. There are four categories of phonetic study that are of particular interest to the SLP:

Physiological Phonetics—this discipline is concerned with how the speech organs work together to produce speech. Understanding Physiological Phonetics is clearly vital to the SLP.

Acoustic Phonetics—this specialty is related to the physical properties of speech sounds.

Perceptual Phonetics—this field is involved in understanding how people make sense of the speech sounds they hear.

Clinical Phonetics— this branch focuses on how SLPs use knowledge of phonetics to diagnose and remediate unintelligible speech.

TERMS YOU SHOULD KNOW

Phonetics is a vital tool for the SLP in the management of speech sound disorders, because it not only helps the SLP document how speech is actually produced, it also provides a written and permanent record of what was uttered. This visual documentation is used in the analysis of speech sound disorders and helps with the tracking of client progress. To use phonetics and phonology to their full extent, you will first need to learn some important terms that provide the foundation for the material presented in this text. Each new concept is presented along with exercises designed to facilitate your understanding of this new material.

VOWELS AND CONSONANTS

There are two familiar classifications for speech sounds, vowels and consonants. Consonants are made with some degree of constriction within the vocal tract, while vowels, on the other hand, are produced with a relatively unobstructed vocal tract. Consonants provide intelligibility to our utterances while vowels provide the power. This text will introduce these vital sounds that make up our speech. Phonetic transcription using IPA will also be a focus. Students often feel that IPA is like learning a "new language." You will be introduced to unique symbols to represent vowels and consonants as you learn to transcribe the IPA.

ENGLISH ORTHOGRAPHY

Orthography is a writing system. English orthography is not sufficient for the SLP. There are 26 orthographic letters (graphemes) in English to represent approximately 44 phonemes. Of the 26 letters of the alphabet, three are unnecessary (Van Riper & Smith, 1979). The letter *c* most often represents the *k* sound as in *cat,* or the *s* sound as in *cease*; therefore, the letter c is not needed. The letter *x* is actually two different speech sounds *ks* as in box, which is transcribed */baks/.* Lastly, the q as in *queen* is not needed because it also represents two sounds *kw* as in *queen* which is transcribed */kwin/.* There are a number of IPA symbols representing consonants that will be familiar, because they are the same as orthographic consonants. They are:

p as in *pup* = /p /	*f as* in *food* = /f/
b as in *boy* = /b/	*v* as in *vent* = /v/
t as in *tea* = /t/	*h* as in *hot* = /h/
d as in *dog* = /d/	*n* as in *no* = /n/
k as in *king* = /k/	*m* as in *mom* = /m/
g as in *gift* = /g/	*r* as in *run* = /r/
s as *say* = /s/	*l* as in *lake* = /l/
z as in *zoo* = /z/	*w* as in *wait* = /w/

The following represents IPA consonants that may be unfamiliar:

sh as in *shut* = /ʃ/	*ch* as in *chip* =/ʧ/	*j* as in *juice* = /ʤ/
y as in *yuck* = /j/	*zh* as in *pleasure* = /ʒ/	
ng as in *sing* = /ŋ/	*th* as in *bath* =/θ/	*th* as in *bathe* = /ð/

Graphemes

A grapheme is an orthographic letter. Graphemes do not provide an adequate means of characterizing the phonological structure of words, because graphemes and speech sounds (phonemes) do not have a one-to-one representation. For example, the word *though* is spelled using six graphemes to represent only two phonemes :/ðo/.

Students learning the IPA often have difficulty "disregarding" the spelling of words when determining what speech sounds (phonemes) are used in the production of words. There are many different reasons that this is a difficult task. The presence of "silent" letters is one such reason. For example, the word *bomb* is composed of four graphemes: *b-o-m-b*, but when the word is spoken aloud with each speech sound segmented, it is clear that the word consists of just three phonemes: *b-o-m* /bɑm/. That is because the final *b* in *bomb* is a silent grapheme.

Identify the *silent* letter(s).

Ex. Dumb → "b"

Exercise 1.1 Identify the silent consonant graphemes in the following words:

Wrap	Wednesday	Lamb	Thumb
Subtle	Gnome	Psychic	Receipt
Autumn	Assign	Cologne	Knee
Honest	Knife	Yolk	Island
Ballet	Gnat	Answer	Psalm

Phones and Phonemes

A wide variety of sounds, called phones, comprises the many languages spoken throughout the world. A phone is any sound that can be produced by the human vocal tract (O'Grady, Archibald, Aronoff & Rees-Miller, 2001). A "raspberry," a sound made by sticking the tongue between the rounded lips and blowing, is a phone; clicking your tongue to indicate disapproval of someone's behavior is also a phone, as is the speech sound */k/* in the word *key*. In all the above examples, sounds are being produced by the vocal tract. A phoneme is a family of phones or speech sounds and is the smallest linguistic unit of language that distinguishes words from each other (Van Riper & Smith, 1979). When produced in isolation, phonemes are not meaningful, but when combined with other phonemes, they create words. For example, the words *bat* and *pat* are "minimal pairs," meaning they differ by just one speech sound. It is the first phoneme in each word that differentiates the two words and signals the meaning difference. No phoneme will be produced in the same way each time it is articulated, because all speech sounds influence the sounds next to them. MacKay (1987) suggested that the concept of the phoneme is abstract, because it is not a single, unchanging unit. Rather than static productions, in order to make speech flow, slight adjustments are made in the way speech sounds are produced, thereby creating allophones (allophones will be discussed in the next section). This makes speech more efficient and more effective as a means of communication.

It can be a difficult task to attune to the individual sounds in a word, because the human brain evolved to focus on the message being communicated and not the individual phonemes comprising the message. The first exercise is designed to help you focus on phonemes that make up words, rather than the letters used to spell them.

For the exercise below, count the number of graphemes used in the spelling of the word, then say the word aloud and count the number of phonemes that are used by segmenting each individual speech sound.

Exercise 1.2 Identify the number of graphemes (G) and phonemes (P) in words:

Orthographic	# of G	# of P	Orthographic	# of G	# of P
Chip	4	3	Sawed		
Hat			Mix		
Clap			Bring		
Face			Write		
Run			Know		
Does			Loose		
Stash			Throat		
Wrinkle			Tea		
That			Thorough		
Back			Quack		

Allophones

Allophones are variations of phonemes (Shriberg & Kent, 1995). Phonemes are produced in the presence of other phonemes, which result in differences in how they are articulated. The influence that phonemes have on each other when produced in strings is known as **coarticulation**, which will be discussed in Chapter 8. Allophones of the same phoneme are phonetically similar and share phonetic features. They will be so similar that most speakers will not distinguish a difference. Phonemes are thought to be a group of allophones that are all perceived in the identical manner (Parker & Riley, 2010). Say the word *sun*. What are your lips doing as you pronounce the *s*? Now say the word *construe*, and note what your lips do while producing the *s*. Are they neutral for the production of *sun* and rounded for *construe*? The reason for the lips rounding on the *s* in *construe* and not *sun* is due to the presence of the rounded vowel */u/* at the end of the word *construe*. It changes the way in which the *s* is produced, causing it to be produced with lip-rounding, which is not typical for the *s* phoneme. This rounded *s* is an allophonic variation of the phoneme *s*.

Morphemes

Words make up a lexicon, a speaker's mental dictionary, and unlike the phonemes and syllables that comprise them, words carry meaning. Words are the building blocks for forming sentences, and they are the foundation upon which language is built. Morphology is the linguistic rule system for the formation of words and word structure.

Linguists define **words** as the smallest **free forms** found in a language (O'Grady, Archibald, Aronoff & Rees-Miller, 2001). Words are not dependent on a fixed position in regard to neighboring elements; they can even appear in isolation. Consider the word *cats*. It is a free form and, thus, a word, because it can occur in isolation, and even when it is part of a sentence, it isn't attached to anything else and can appear in varying positions within a sentence. Sometimes nouns occur before verbs as in "*Cats* hate baths," and sometimes they follow verbs as in "Dogs hate *cats*." However, the plural marker *–s* in the word *cats* cannot appear in isolation and cannot be separated from the noun.

A morpheme is the smallest unit that signals a semantic interpretation (O'Grady, Archibald, Aronoff & Rees-Miller, 2001). A morpheme can be a word by itself, such as the word *cat,* which is composed of one morpheme. Its semantic interpretation is that it is a furry animal that drinks milk and says, "Meow." Two morphemes comprise the word *cats*. The plural marker *–s* signals that there is more than one furry animal that drinks milk and says, "Meow." *Cat* is a **free morpheme**, because it can appear in isolation and make sense. The plural marker *-s* is a **bound morpheme**, because it must be attached to a free morpheme to convey information concerning meaning or function. Another example illustrating free and bound morphemes is the word *walked*. *Walk* is a free morpheme, because it can stand alone and have meaning, i.e., to put one foot in front of the other. The tense marker *–ed* is a bound morpheme, because it must be attached to the free morpheme to convey its meaning, i.e., action that happened in the past. *Samantha's* is another example of free and bound morphemes. *Samantha*, a free morpheme, indicates (in this example) my dog, and the possessive marker *–'s* is a bound morpheme indicating something that belongs to her, such as her chew bone.

Exercise 1.3 Identify number of morphemes:

Orthographic	Morphemes	Number	Orthographic	Morphemes	Number
Bats	Bat-s	2	Slices		

Ran			Boyishness		
Walking			Downtown		
It's			Grapes		
Higher			Gentleman		
Around			Water		
Rebound			Drawing		
Basketball			Paints		
Unhappiest			Jeff's		
Dogs			Haircut		

Consonant Singletons

A **consonant singleton** is a single consonant phoneme appearing before or after a vowel. For example, in the word *block* /blɑk/, the /k/ is a singleton consonant, because it appears by itself after the vowel. The /bl/ is a **consonant cluster**, which will be discussed next.

Consonant Clusters or Blends

A **consonant cluster**, also called a **consonant blend**, is a combination of two, three, or four consonant letters in consecutive order with each producing a sound. For example, the *pr* in *pray* are both pronounced, as are the *spl* in *split*. Although extremely rare, four consonant phonemes can be combined in the final positions of words, for example *texts* /tɛksts/.

Exercise 1.4 Underline the consonant cluster:

Ex. Split → Split

Splash	Squid	Spill	Cluster	Black
Desk	Swing	Plate	Spring	Stripe
Spray	Plaster	Spots	Clasp	Blast
Queen	Mask	Chest	Glow	Scallop

Digraphs

A digraph is composed of two different graphemes representing one phoneme. Common digraphs in English include *th* /Θ/as in *thumb*, *sh* /ʃ/ as in *shut*, *ng* /ŋ/as in *sing*, and *ch* /ʧ/ as in *church*. Understanding that two letters represent only one speech sound can be tricky for students at first. The following exercise will help you become a pro at spotting digraphs.

Exercise 1.5 Underline the digraph in each word:

Ex. shoot → "shoot"

hush	sh	ships	
growth		switch	
thrush		philosophy	
church		laughing	
trash		swing	

phone		shout	
beach		digraph	
pocket		whale	
which		mouth	
clock		bridge	

Cognates

Cognates are pairs of phonemes that differ only by the feature of **voicing**, i.e., they are produced in the same place within the oral cavity using the same articulators in the same way or manner. There are eight pairs of cognates in English (Singh & Singh, 2006). An example of a pair of cognates is /p/ as in pit and /b/ as in bit. Both of these phonemes are made by "stopping" the air (manner) with the two lips (place). Touch your larynx with your fingers as you say the /b/ sound. Did you feel vibrations? The vibrations are the vocal fold vibrating thus producing the voicing element for the /b/. Try again with /p/. You didn't feel any vibrations that time, did you? That's because the /p/ is a voiceless sound and is produced without vocal fold vibration.

Minimal Pairs

Minimal pairs are two words differing by only one phoneme. Minimal pairs can vary by either consonants or vowels. For example:

1. pat /pæt/ and bat /bæt/ are minimal pairs, because they differ by the first phoneme, which is a consonant.
2. pit /pɪt/ and pat /pæt/ are minimal pairs, because they differ by the vowel.
3. pot /pɑt/ and pod /pɑd/ are minimal pairs, because they differ by the final phoneme, which is a consonant.

Diacritics

One of the primary advantages of using the IPA is that it affords SLPs a mechanism for representing speech sounds as they are heard, rather than how they are spelled. **Diacritics,** unique markings that denote variations in the production of phonemes, are particularly useful when transcribing disordered speech and will be discussed at length in Chapter 9. Diacritics are used to signify allophonic variations of diverse speakers and dialects (Van Riper & Smith, 1979). SLPs use both broad and narrow transcription when transcribing a client's speech. There are important differences between the two types of transcription.

Broad Transcription (also called *phonemic transcription)*: the process of using IPA symbols to represent speech sounds. Broad transcription makes use of virgules / / to indicate that the symbols contained within the virgules are IPA symbols (Van Riper & Smith, 1979).

Narrow Transcription (also called *phonetic transcription*): the process of using IPA symbols to represent speech as it was actually spoken. Narrow transcription deals with allophonic variations and uses diacritic markings to show how sounds are produced in context. The diacritical marks used in phonetic transcription are imperative when transcribing disordered speech. Phonetic transcription is also used when transcribing actual speech. Brackets [ ] are used to delineate phonetic (narrow) transcription from phonemic (broad) transcription (Van Riper & Smith, 1979).

SYLLABLES AND SOUND

Syllables and phonemes are considered **segmental units** of speech (Van Riper & Smith, 1979). Phonemes comprise syllables, and every syllable must consist of at least a vowel sound. The vowel will function as the **nucleus**, or peak, of the syllable. The **nucleus** (vowel) may be surrounded by one or more consonants. When a syllable contains a consonant preceding the vowel, this is known as the syllable **onset** (or releasing consonant). Any consonant sound following the vowel is known as the **coda** (or arresting consonant). In the word *cat* /kæt/, the /k/ precedes the **nucleus** /æ/, so it is the syllable **onset**; the /t/ follows the vowel, making it the syllable **coda** (Edwards & Shriberg, 1983).

Prevocalic

Prevocalic means "before the vowel" and refers to consonants (both singleton and clusters) that precede a vowel sound. In the word *cat* /kæt/, the /k/ comes before the vowel, so it is **prevocalic.**

Intervocalic

Intervocalic refers to consonants appearing between two vowels. In the word *kitten /kɪtɛn/*, the */t/* comes between two vowels, so it is **intervocalic.**

Postvocal

Postvocalic refers to a consonant that comes after a vowel. In the word *cat* /kæt/, the /t/ comes after the vowel, so it is **postvocalic.**

Exercise 1.6 Identify if each consonant is prevocalic, intervocalic, or postvocalic:

*Note that in the first example *ballet,* even though there is a *t* at the end, the *t* is silent; therefore, it would not be considered postvocalic. There are also two *l*'s in *ballet* that represent only one */l/* sound. Say each word aloud.

Orthographic Word	Prevocalic	Intervocalic	Postvocalic
ballet	b	l	
carrot			
hope			
button			
colon			
narrow			
dog			
wagon			
boat			
cook			

Syllables can also be characterized as either open or closed (Yavas, 2006). An **open** syllable is one that ends in a vowel sound (no coda is present). A **closed** syllable is one that ends in a consonant sound (has a coda). For example, the word *bough /baʊ/* ends in a diphthong; therefore, it is considered an open syllable even though it ends in the orthographic letters *gh*. The word bat /bæt/ ends in the phoneme /t/; therefore, it is considered a closed syllable.

Because every syllable must contain a nucleus, the nucleus can also be referred to as a **syllabic.** A syllabic can be a "pure" vowel (monothong) such as /æ/ as in cat /kæt/, or it can be a **diphthong** (two consecutive vowels produced with rapid articulation, thus combining to form a single speech sound). For example, the *oy* in *boy* /bɔɪ/ is a diphthong, because it is composed of the **onglide** /ɔ/ and **offglide** /ɪ/. (Diphthongs will be discussed in greater detail in Chapter 4.) A syllabic can also be a vowel and consonant combination. For example, the *el* /l̩/ sound in *bottle* /bɑtl̩/ is a **syllabic consonant.** (Syllabic consonants will be addressed in Chapter 8.)

Consonants can be added to the vowel nucleus to form various syllable shapes. Throughout this text, for each syllable shape, *V* will represent the vowel nucleus, and *C* will represent a consonant.

This chart represents different syllable shapes in English and gives an example of each. Keep in mind that syllable shapes are dependent on phonemes, not orthographic letters.

Syllables	**IPA**	**Orthographic**
Open		
V	/aɪ/	I
CV	/mi/	me
CCV	/ste/	stay
CCCV	/stre/	stray
Closed		
VC	/ɔn/	on
VCC	/ɛnd/	end

VCCC	/æsks/	ends
CVC	/kæn/	can
CVCC	/bænd/	band
CVCCC	/bɛnds/	bends
CVCCCC	/sɪksθs/	sixths
CCVC	/dræg/	drag
CCVCC	/spʌndʒ/	sponge
CCVCCC	/blɛndz/	blends
CCCVC	/striŋ/	string
CCCVCC	/sprɪnt/	sprint
CCCVCCCC	/skræmblz/	scrambles

Exercise 1.7 Identify the number of syllables:

Orthographic	Identify syllables	Number of Syllables
popcorn	pop-corn	2

(*Continued*)

night		
you		
thinking		
football		
elements		
tour		
directions		
super		
jargon		
superstition		
aardvark		
trampoline		
dig		
segments		
earlobe		

scramble		
down		
up		
I		

CONCLUSION

Speech-language pathologists require a written record of speech to diagnose, treat, and track the progress of speech disorders. Orthography is inadequate for this task due to the many inconsistencies in the English language and alphabet; however, the IPA combined with knowledge of phonology and phonetics provide the perfect tools to help the SLP manage speech disorders.

This chapter's presentation of terms and concepts will aid in your understanding of the task ahead—becoming a skilled transcriber, assessor, and analyzer of speech. Learning these concepts and the ones presented later might seem like a daunting task, but they provide the foundation for skills that will be invaluable to you as an SLP.

IMAGE CREDIT

- Fig 1.1: Copyright © International Phonetic Association (CC BY-SA 3.0) at https://en.wikipedia.org/wiki/File:The_International_Phonetic_Alphabet_(revised_to_2015).pdf.

CHAPTER

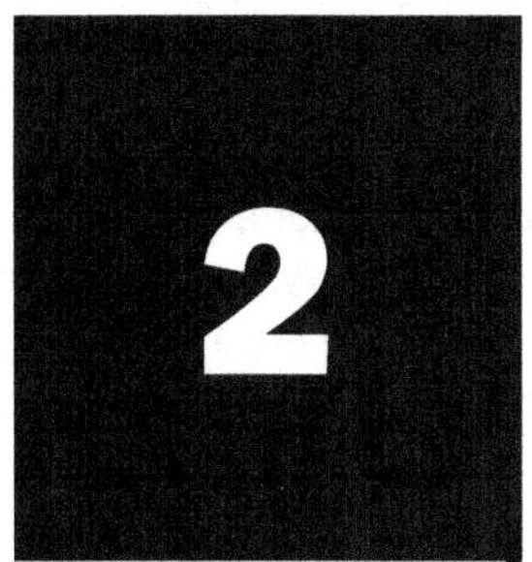

We do not know when or why humans began to produce vocalizations now known as speech, but this complex feat has helped catapult the species to remarkable achievements. Speech is the foundation on which human language developed, and it enables abstract thought, the planning and implementation of social order, and the ability to pass knowledge to future generations.

HOW SPEECH IS PRODUCED

The structures used to generate speech all have primary biological functions that are vital to survival. At some point during evolution, humans requisitioned four major biological systems for speech production purposes. These four systems are the respiration system, the phonation system, the resonation system, and the articulation system. Muscles in the abdomen, chest, neck, and head work together in the production of speech. Although these systems and the production of speech are discussed in this chapter in a linear fashion, it is important to understand that they work synergistically to produce speech.

All speech begins with intent, and all physical movement to make intent happen originates and is mediated by the central nervous system (CNS), which is composed of the brain and spinal cord (La Pointe, 2011). Whether it is a warning to a child not to dart out into traffic or a request to a friend to go to a movie, the CNS not only receives input from the body and the environment, but it also organizes all activity of the body. The sensation that one is hot is obtained from the CNS; the idea and physical movements associated with turning on the air conditioning is also coordinated by the CNS.

How communicative intentions become verbal is the outcome of primarily biological mechanisms working in concert in a connected sequence to create the rapidly changing modifications of the airstream that results in sounds known as speech. Respiration is the first system discussed in this chapter. Its primary function is to keep the body alive by providing oxygen to the blood. For the production of speech, it provides the power source—air.

THE RESPIRATION SYSTEM

The act of breathing in (inhalation) and breathing out (exhalation) is called respiration and is vital to survival. Exhaled air is what makes speech possible, for speech is simply shaped air (West & Kantner, 1941). Sometimes the shaped air will be voiced, and sometimes it will have no voicing component. (Voiced and voiceless sounds will be discussed later in the phonation section in this chapter). The respiratory system is responsible for the oxygen/carbon dioxide exchange that provides life. Air is breathed in through the nose or the mouth with these two airways meeting at the pharynx (throat), which is located at the back of the mouth and is used for both digestion and respiration. The pharynx divides into two paths—one path, the trachea (windpipe), carries air to the lungs, and the other path, the esophagus, carries food and drink to be used by the digestive system. The epiglottis (a small flap of tissue) covers the trachea when swallowing occurs. The larynx (voice box) is a boney structure that sits at the top of the trachea and protects the vocal folds. The vocal folds close (adduct) when swallowing occurs. This closing action, along with action from the epiglottis, stops food and liquid from going into the lungs. The trachea extends downward from the bottom of the larynx and is lined by stiff rings of cartilage, which keep it open. The trachea is divided into two branches with each branch leading to one of the lungs. In the lungs, each branch of the trachea continues to divide into smaller and finer branches, called bronchi. This "branching" is similar to a tree. The smallest divisions of the bronchi are called bronchioles, which end in air sacs called alveoli. There are hundreds of millions of alveoli in each lung, and this is where the body swaps oxygen with carbon dioxide gasses.

Humans speak on egressed or exhaled air. It is this exhaled air that supplies the initial energy source that makes speech possible. The amount of air required for different speaking tasks varies. During normal respiration, involving no speaking or physical exertion, the exhalation rate versus inhalation rate is roughly 50/50. Speech requires a 1/10 ratio for inhalation to exhalation and can be even greater depending upon the task (Seikel, Drumright, and Seikel 2013). Singers, for example, require a much longer exhalation period versus inhalation period. Depending on the task, more extended exhalation periods are needed to sustain the air support necessary for each speaking situation. Whether one is cheerleading, performing in a play, singing in the choir, or just talking quietly with a friend, the amount of air required and the period of exhalation will differ. Respiration for speech production also differs from respiration for life support in that it includes quick intakes of air and metered exhalations (Seikel, Drumright, and Seikel 2013).

The major players of inhalation are the dome-shaped diaphragm, the lungs, the trachea, the external intercostal muscles, and the costal elevator muscles of the thorax (rib cage). Breathing starts with the contraction of the largest muscle of respiration, the diaphragm. As the diaphragm contracts, the external intercostal muscles and costal elevator muscles contract, causing the thoracic cavity to expand. The lungs fill with air because of a change in air pressure. There is a negative pressure inside the lungs relative to the atmospheric pressure. Equalization of this pressure is desperately sought, which will cause air to be sucked in via the mouth and/or nose. The lungs, because they are elastic, will expand (West & Kantner, 1941).

A good way to understand the process of respiration is to think about the steps needed to breathe. First, depress the diaphragm. The stomach will bulge out as the diaphragm flattens. It may be necessary to lie on the floor with a book on the stomach to get a good picture of the movement of the diaphragm. As inhalation and exhalation occur, the book should rise and fall. Also, note the feeling of the external intercostal muscles and the costal elevator muscles as they contract. Feel these muscles rotating the ribs outward. Hold the breath stream until the urge to exhale becomes unbearable. The exhalation process is a combination of three basic steps. First, the muscles of inhalation will relax. Feel the diaphragm returning to its normal position and the external intercostal muscles and costal elevator muscles relaxing so that the ribs go back to their starting position. When the muscles responsible for inhalation relax, the lungs return to their original size and shape. Second, gravity plays a role. When positioned either sitting or standing erect, gravity will act on the ribs to pull them back to their starting point. And last, the cartilage and lung tissue are elastic, and just like a rubber band, they will return to their original position. Together, these three properties will result in air being expelled from the lungs at which point it enters the larynx. As mentioned earlier, the amount of air expelled will be different depending on the type of activity in which one is engaged. Whether one is breathing quietly, playing sports, speaking, or singing, air is vital for all of these tasks. Pushing more air out of the lungs will result in increased loudness.

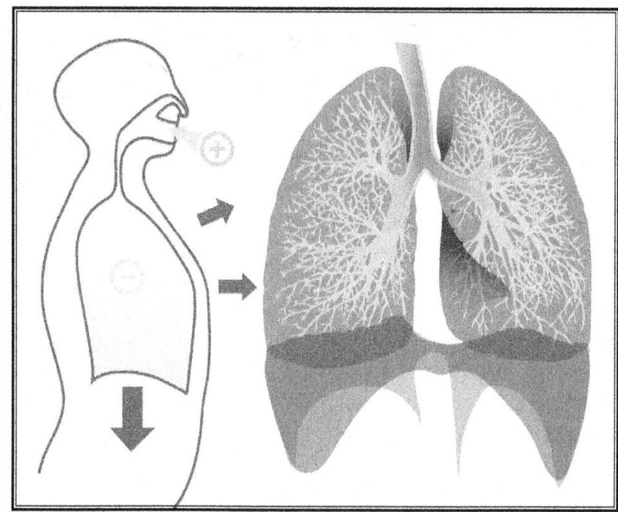

Fig. 2.1 Lungs

Air is the power source for speech, so the more efficiently one breathes, the better and more diverse one's speaking needs will be. Of the three basic types of breathing— clavicular, thoracic, and diaphragmatic—diaphragmatic breathing produces the best breath support for speech production. Clavicular breathing provides the least. Try out clavicular breathing, and it will quickly be evident why it is not a good option for speech production. Clavicular breathing expands the thorax by contracting the sternum. This does not increase the thorax sufficiently. Try clavicular breathing out now by concentrating on increasing the thorax by contraction of the sternum. Are you dizzy yet? It's clear how this would not be an adequate option for speech production. Breath support for typical speaking situations is usually a combination of thoracic and diaphragmatic breathing. It's important for speech-language pathologists (SLPs) to understand the best way to breathe for speech production, because speech is simply shaped air.

Major Structures of the Respiration System:

Diaphragm: This dome-shaped muscle separates the abdominal cavity from the thoracic cavity. It is also the main muscle of inspiration. A downward motion of the diaphragm occurs when the radiating fibers of the diaphragm pull on the central tendon. When the diaphragm contracts, it allows the thoracic cavity to increase, creating space so that the lungs can expand when they fill with air. The process of inhalation and exhalation occurs roughly 12 times per minute during normal breathing for an adult.

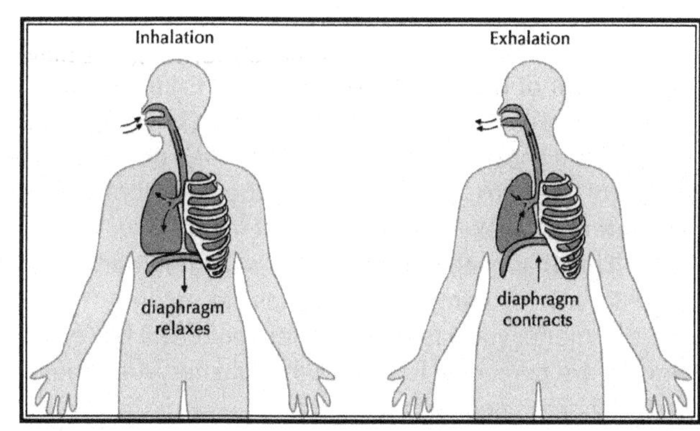

Fig 2.2: Diaphragm

External Intercostal: These 11 muscles are located between the 12 ribs of the thorax (Seikel, Drumright, and Seikel 2013) are considered accessory muscles of inhalation, and they allow the ribs to move in unity to elevate the entire rib cage (Perkins & Kent, 1986). Elevating the rib cage enlarges the transverse dimension. The external intercostal muscles usually aren't engaged for quiet breathing, but the contraction of these muscles significantly increases the amount of air needed to produce speech.

Lungs: These elastic cone-shaped organs are housed in the thoracic cavity, which supports them with muscle and bone. Enlarging the rib cage causes the lungs to fill with air. The air enters and escapes the lungs through the bronchial tree and upper respiratory passageway (Perkins & Kent, 1986).

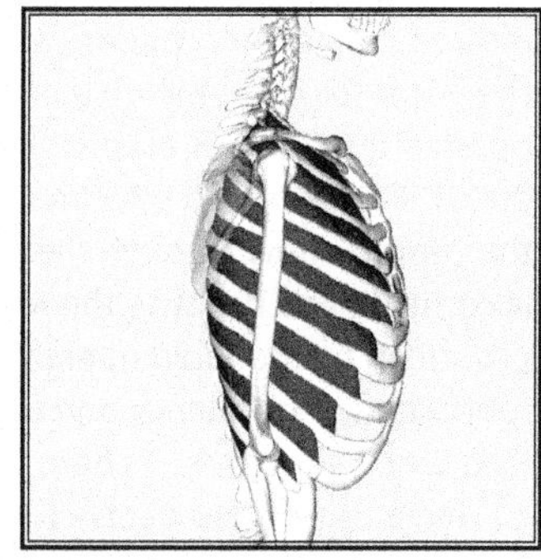

Fig 2.3: External Intercostals

THE PHONATION SYSTEM

Normal breathing produces an inaudible breath stream, so, for speech to happen, a sound source must be added. Speech would not be possible without a voicing component, because all vowel sounds are voiced, and many of the consonants are voiced as well. The phonation system, like the respiration system, not only allows for speech production, but also plays a primary role in supporting life. The major player of the phonation system is the larynx, which houses the vocal folds and acts as a valve for the airflow exiting the lungs. The vocal folds are the vibrating element and, thus, the source of phonation.

The larynx, constructed of muscles and cartilage, moves up and down during speaking and swallowing (MacKay & MacKay, 1987). The vocal folds are elastic tissue composed mainly of muscle. They extend from the thyroid cartilage at the front to the arytenoid cartilages at the back. Each of the vocal folds attaches to a separate arytenoid cartilage. The space between the vocal folds is called the glottis. When the arytenoids come together as a result of muscle contraction, the vocal folds adduct (close). This allows for the impounding of air in the thoracic cavity. This impounded air allows for a variety of life-sustaining tasks, such as lifting heavy objects, defecating, giving birth, and safely swallowing food and drinks without choking. For speech production purposes, the impounded air causes the vocal folds to vibrate, providing the phonation that permits the production of voiced speech sounds. If we were unable to produce voicing, humans would not be able to make the vowel sounds and voiced consonants that make speech possible. When breathing, the vocal folds are abducted, meaning they are open, revealing the glottis. Air enters and escapes via the glottis during quiet breathing.

When talking, the vocal folds close (adduct), causing air pressure to build up below them (subglottal pressure). Eventually, this pressure becomes so great that it blows the vocal folds apart, releasing a puff of compressed air. The folds return to their starting position, and once again, pressure builds up, a puff of compressed air is released, and the cycle repeats. The vibrating vocal folds rhythmically open and close, interrupting the steady stream of air. The release of this series of puffs of compressed air is the source of the sound known as "voice." The number of these "cycles" per second is known as fundamental frequency (Seikel, Drumright, & Seikel 2013), which is expressed in units called hertz (Hz). Fundamental frequency is perceived as vocal "pitch." The size and mass of the vocal folds determine the range of frequencies for a given speaker's voice. Adjusting the tension and length of the folds, which will cause them to vibrate at different rates, can alter pitch. Pitch is changed (varying intonation) to make speech more interesting. Our vocal folds typically vibrate between 80 and 500 Hz while we are talking (Raphael, Borden, & Harris, 2007). Men naturally have thicker vocal folds with more mass that vibrate more slowly, resulting in fewer cycles per second. That is the reason a man's pitch is perceived as being lower. The average male's vocal folds vibrate at about 125 Hz (cycles per second), the average female's at about 220 Hz; thus, women are perceived to have higher pitches. And, the act of singing can require a vocal fold vibration of as much as 1,200 cycles per second!

Speech is a complex tone meaning it contains a wide range of frequencies, not just the fundamental frequency (Seikel, Drumright, & Seikel 2013). This is due to the way in which the vocal folds vibrate. The folds open from the bottom to the top and from the back to the front in a wave motion that is called the "mucosal wave." This waving motion results in frequencies other than just the fundamental frequency being produced by the vocal folds. When the vocal folds are blown apart and release a puff of air, they are sucked back together more quickly than they opened due to their elasticity and an aerodynamic principle called the Bernoulli Effect (Pena-Brooks & Hegde, 2000). The Bernoulli Effect causes the folds to be sucked back together at a faster rate than they opened, because the rapid airflow through the glottis causes a simultaneous drop in air pressure. Because the vocal fold movement is complex and because the folds open more slowly than they close, more than the fundamental frequency is produced by the rapid opening and closing of the glottis. The result is a complex harmonic sound containing the fundamental frequency and the harmonics or "overtones." The harmonic released is a multiple of the fundamental frequency. Energy, in its harmonic component, declines as frequency increases. This rate of decline in energy is 12 decibels (dB) per octave (doubling in frequency). Harmonics provide richness to the voice (Seikel, Drumright, & Seikel 2013). To understand the contribution of harmonics to the human voice, consider the two music icons Barry White and Barry Gibb. Barry White's low pitch coupled with extensive harmonics produced his distinctive bass-baritone voice that made him a soul music legend. Barry Gibb's signature falsetto, on the other hand, propelled his band, the Bee Gees, to stardom during the disco era. The laryngeal adjustments needed to produce Gibb's iconic style of singing resulted in a higher pitch with far fewer harmonics. Search the Internet to see and hear these artists perform. By comparing the two performances, the differences of the complex tone known as speech becomes apparent.

At the point of phonation, the fundamental frequency and the harmonics do not sound like a human voice. Instead, this spectrum from the glottis sounds like a "buzz," which is referred to as the "laryngeal tone." This complex tone must go through resonation, which causes certain components to be amplified and other components to be dampened before it will sound like speech.

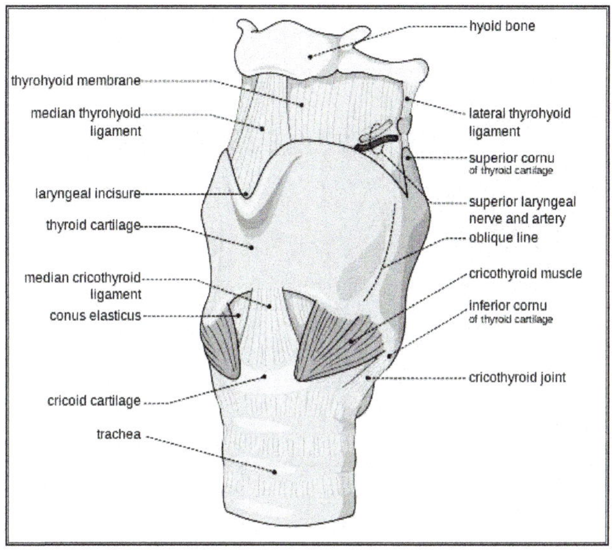

Fig. 2.4: Larynx

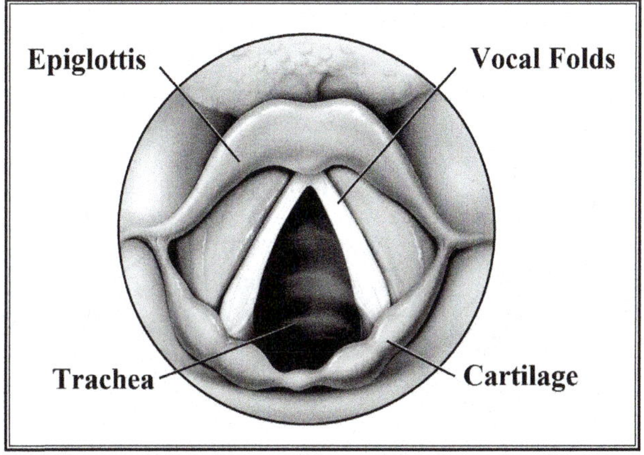

Fig. 2.5: Vocal Fold

Major Structures of Phonation:

Larynx: This structure composed of five cartilages, muscles, membranes, and connective ligaments houses the vocal folds.

Vocal Folds: These mucous-covered, elastic folds are made up of the thyroarytenoid muscles of the larynx and vocal ligaments and provide the vibrating element for speech. Tensing the vocal folds makes them vibrate faster, producing an increase in pitch.

THE RESONATION SYSTEM

The process by which the voiced breath stream (laryngeal tone) is modified to enhance and dampen certain frequency components is known as resonation. A resonator must be closed at one end and opened at the other end. The vocal tract (oral, nasal, and pharyngeal cavities) serves as our resonator—it is opened at the mouth and closed when the vocal folds are adducted (closed). Speech is a complex sound that contains two types of frequencies. The first, as discussed earlier, is the fundamental frequency, which is the result of vocal fold vibration. The second type of frequency is the formant frequency, which relates to vocal tract configuration. Formants are a natural mode of vibration of the vocal tract. There are an infinite number of formants, but only three are needed to distinguish vowels. Formants don't supply energy; they only modify energy from phonation. Our resonator increases the intensity of certain frequencies of the sounds coming from the larynx and reduces the intensity of others, depending on the way it is shaped. Movements of the tongue, lips, jaw, and velum make it possible to alter the shape of the vocal tract and, thus, generate different speech sounds. Depending upon the shape of the vocal tract, certain parts or frequencies of the complex sound produced by phonation will be selectively amplified. It is at this point that a distinct sound, recognized as a human voice, can be perceived.

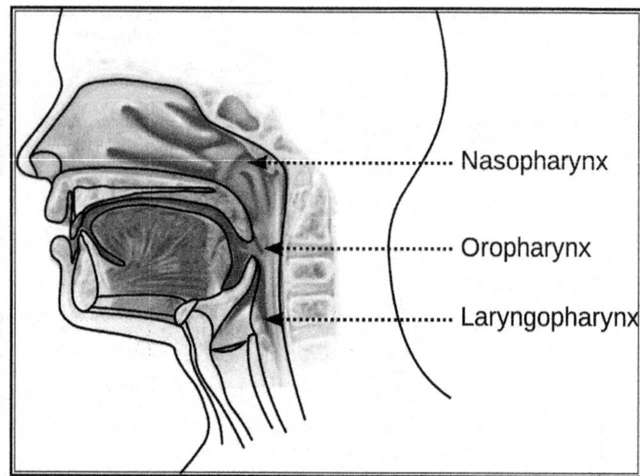

Fig. 2.6: Vocal Tract

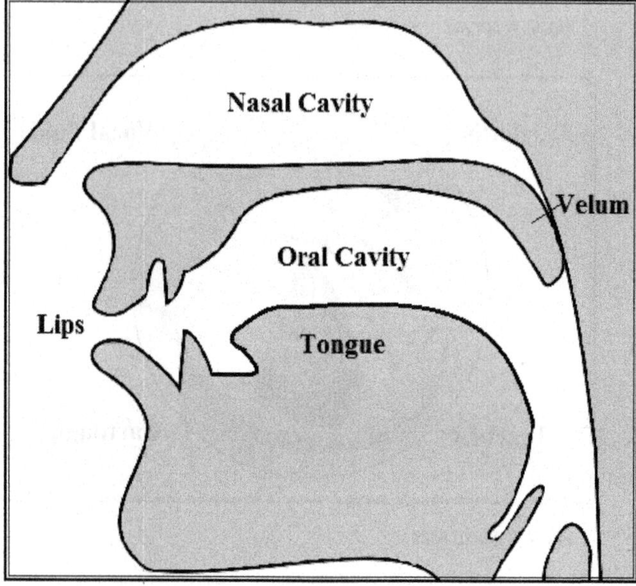

Fig. 2.7: Pharynx

A process known as velopharyngeal closure is necessary for the production of oral speech sounds. This vital act is accomplished by the velum closing against the back of the throat, thereby directing the airflow into the oral cavity. If the velum remains in a relaxed position, the airflow will primarily be directed into the nasal cavity allowing for the production of nasal speech sounds.

Major Structures of Resonation:

Vocal Tract: The vocal tract is a structure lying above the larynx that resembles an intricately shaped "tube" that can be altered by moving the tongue, lips, velum, and other parts of the tract. These movements modify its acoustic properties, thereby allowing for the production of different speech sounds. The oral, nasal, and pharyngeal cavities comprise this very important tube that helps shape the voiced and unvoiced air leaving the larynx into speech sounds.

Pharynx: Located at the root of the tongue and extending downward to the esophagus, the human pharynx is larger than that of other primates due to a lowered larynx. The larger pharynx is crucial to the production of speech, because it enhances the lower resonances needed for vowel production. The pharynx is divided into three distinct sections.

Laryngopharynx: This is the section of the pharynx that joins the larynx.

Nasopharynx: This part of the pharynx is adjacent to the posterior portion of the nasal cavity. The Eustachian tubes, crucial to the equalization of changes in air pressure, connect the nasopharynx with the middle ear mechanism.

Oropharynx: This portion of the pharynx is adjacent to the posterior section of the oral cavity.

THE ARTICULATION SYSTEM

Finally, the articulation system is crucial for speech sound production. The oral cavity is the point of exit for most of the sounds, and alterations of the shape of the cavity is a vital aspect of resonance. The oral cavity also houses the major articulators, including the lips, teeth, alveolar ridge, hard palate, velum, and the tongue (Pena-Brooks & Hegde, 2000). Articulation happens when two or more of the articulators change the manner of airflow. The articulation system also serves as the sound source for voiceless consonants. The air from the lungs is set into motion within the oral cavity by adjustments of the articulators, which produces the "sound" we hear for the voiceless consonants.

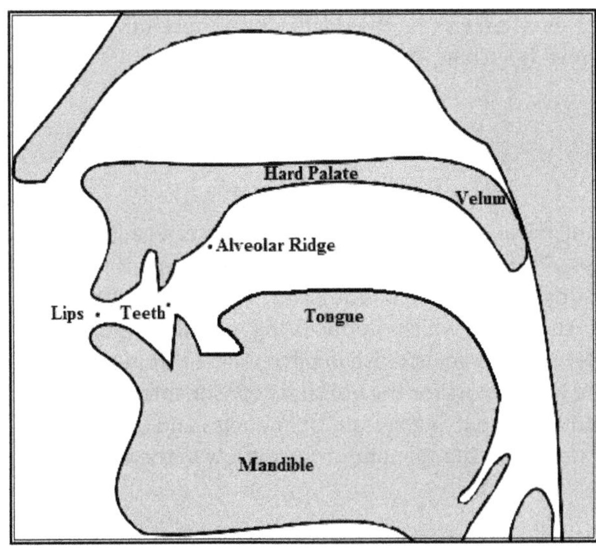

Fig. 2.8: Articulation System

Major Structures of the Articulation System:

Lips: The lips are made up of muscle, the main one being the orbicularis oris, and other tissues. The muscles of the lips give them a wide range of mobility, allowing them to perform the many movements needed not only for eating, but for producing speech sounds, as well. The lips are described in terms of "roundness" for vowel production and help shape the oral cavity to produce different vowels. "Labial' speech sounds, those which engage the lips, are also made possible and include /p/, /m/, and /w/ to name a few.

Teeth: Adults have 32 teeth (16 upper and 16 lower). The teeth are embedded within the upper and lower jaw. The teeth provide the crucial biological function of biting and chewing food. The teeth serve as an immobile articulator with which the tongue can make contact to produce the "lingua-dental" sounds (the voiced and voiceless "th") or help channel the flow of air in the production of certain sounds, such as /s/.

Hard Palate: The hard palate is a boney structure that makes up the roof of the oral cavity and serves as the floor of the nasal cavity. It acts as a barrier between the two cavities preventing food and liquids from entering the nasal cavity. It also serves as an immobile articulator and makes the production of "palatal" speech sounds such as "sh" and "ch" possible.

Alveolar Ridge: This raised ridge runs from side to side toward the anterior of the hard palate and is located just behind the upper teeth. It is critical to the production of "alveolar" speech sounds, such as /t/ and /l/.

Velum (Soft Palate): The velum is composed of muscles and other soft tissues and is located posterior to the hard palate. The velum aids in both swallowing and speech production, because it is made of a number of muscles and can move. The velum joins or separates the oral and nasal cavities, allowing air to pass through the oral cavity, the nasal cavity, or both—it is the velum that is responsible for airflow into either the oral or the nasal cavities. When the velum is at rest, it hangs down into the pharynx, creating a passageway, called the velopharyngeal port, between the oral and nasal cavities. When the velopharyngeal port is open, the oral and nasal cavities are "coupled," and air is free to resonate in both cavities, allowing for the production of the nasal speech sounds /m/, /n/, and *ng,* as in *sing*.

All other speech sounds are "oral" sounds and require that the velum be raised up and back, touching the posterior pharyngeal wall, so the air flows only through the oral cavity. When the back of the tongue makes contact with the velum, the "velar" speech sounds /k/, /g/, and "ng" are produced. It is vital that the velopharyngeal port is closed when swallowing, so that food and drink don't enter the nasal cavity.

Tongue: The tongue, our largest articulator, is a complex of muscles and occupies most of the oral cavity. It is capable of assuming a variety of shapes and positions, and its flexibility and speed of mobility is critical to performing such essential functions as chewing and swallowing. It is also vital to speech production, allowing for vowel and consonant articulation. The tongue is needed to produce "lingual" consonant speech sounds, and its movements also alter the shape of the oral cavity, thus producing different resonance characteristics of the vocal tract, making vowel production possible. In terms of speech production, the tongue is divided into five major sections: the tip, or apex; the blade; the back, or dorsum; the root; and the body.

Mandible: The mandible is the lower jaw, and its movement is instrumental in changing the shape of the oral cavity. It houses the lower teeth and is vital in biting and chewing food. By opening and closing the mandible, we produce different vowel sounds. When you "open wide" such as when visiting the doctor for a check-up, vowel sounds such as "ah" are possible, when you close your jaw, vowels such as "eee" can be made.

CONCLUSION

Speech is the production of sounds by the vocal tract (the oral, nasal, and pharyngeal cavities). It is a complex process that requires the biological systems to work in concert. The power source for speech is air that is moved by the respiratory system. Pushing more air out of the lungs results in increased loudness. Air from the lungs passes through the larynx, causing the adducted (closed) vocal folds to vibrate, which produces the voicing element for all vowels and the voiced consonants. Tensing the vocal folds results in an increase in pitch. The air from the lungs is set into motion within the oral cavity by adjustments of the articulators for the voiceless consonants. The vocal tract provides the resonance quality of speech sounds, selectively amplifying certain frequencies and dampening others. Finally, articulation occurs when two or more articulators alter the manner of the airflow in the oral cavity.

IMAGE CREDITS

- Fig 2.1: "Lungs," https://pixabay.com/en/lungs-diagram-anatomy-body-human-41562/. Copyright in the Public Domain.
- Fig 2.2: Copyright © Siyavula Education (CC by 2.0) at https://www.flickr.com/photos/121935927@N06/13578797865.
- Fig 2.3: Copyright © Anatomography (CC BY-SA 2.1 Japan) at https://commons.wikimedia.org/wiki/File:External_intercostal_muscles_lateral2.png.
- Fig 2.4: Copyright © Olek Remesz (CC BY-SA 2.5) at https://commons.wikimedia.org/wiki/File:Larynx_external_en.svg.
- Fig 2.5: Alan Hoofring, "Larynx Top Fold," https://commons.wikimedia.org/wiki/File:Larynx_(top_view).jpg. Copyright in the Public Domain.
- Fig 2.7: Copyright © Semhur (CC BY-SA 3.0) at https://commons.wikimedia.org/wiki/File:Pharynx_diagram-fr.svg.

CHAPTER

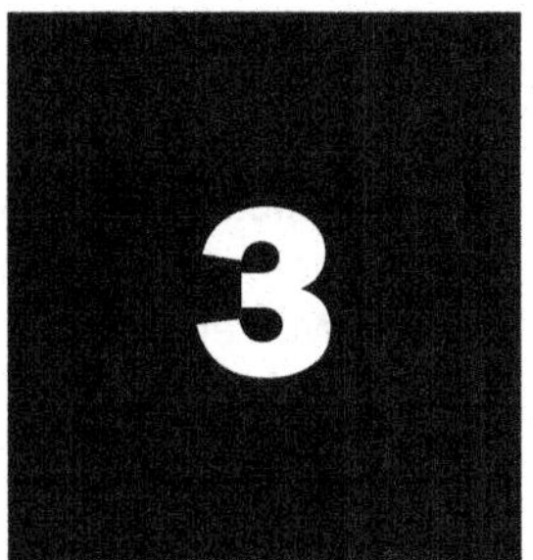

Communication begins at birth. Babies come into the world hard wired to develop the skills necessary to convey their thoughts and feelings to those in charge of their perceived well-being. A child's path to spoken language consists of a series of steps that are relatively consistent across all children, irrespective of their linguistic environment (Stoel-Gammon & Dunn, 1985). Although the human desire to communicate is innate, the rules of a language and the physical structures and movements to produce the sounds known as speech must be developed. The maturational effects of the size and shape of an infant's vocal tract naturally impact phonological acquisition. While a fully formed vocal tract is crucial to the production of adult standard speech, an infant's vocal tract is shorter and flatter and is shaped differently with a shorter pharyngeal cavity and a more gradual bend in the oropharyngeal canal. Also, the larynx is higher, the velopharynx and epiglottis are closer together, and the bulk of the tongue is situated more forward in the oral cavity (Kent & Murray, 1982). As the speech mechanism is developing and growing, children are also acquiring the rules of the phonology of their language. The concurrent motoric and linguistic development will result in a predictable, yet unique, developmental sequence for the perception and production of speech that will be discussed in this chapter. Phonological awareness and its impact on literacy will also be addressed, as well as theories of phonological development.

ACQUISITION OF SPEECH SOUNDS AND PHONOLOGICAL PATTERNS

Phonological development, for the most part, is consistent across children, regardless of native language. Speech perception is the precursor to speech production and involves the recognition of speech sounds from auditory cues (Dirckx, 1997). Research has shown that infants, very early in development, prefer human voices, can localize sounds, and can be conditioned to discriminate between phonemes as young as four days old. Research has further suggested that babies have the innate ability to discriminate differences among phonemes even when those phonemes are not found in their native language, and they have been shown to demonstrate this remarkable feat as young as one month old (Eimas, Siqueland, Jusczyk, and Vigorito, 1971). Between the ages of 6 and 8 months, infants begin to refine discrimination capabilities and can

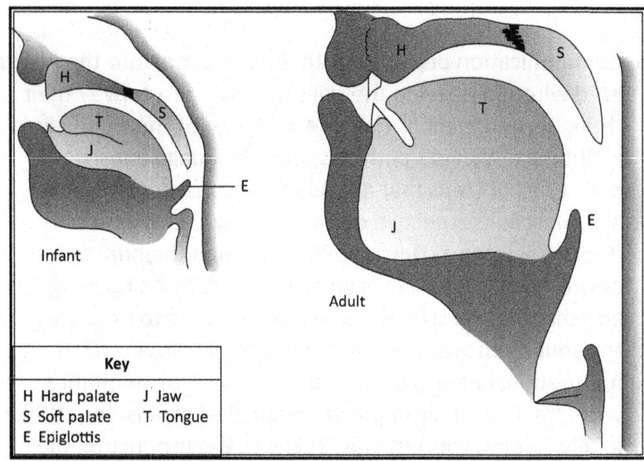

Fig. 3.1: Comparison of Infant and Adult Oral Structures

distinguish between very similar non-native speech sounds; however, around the age of 10 to 12 months, children appear to home in on the "mother tongue" and begin to lose these abilities as they focus on the perception and production of phonemes of their native language (Vihman, 1996; Werker & Polka, 1993).

Regarding speech production, Oller (1980) proposed a series of developmental stages. During prelinguistic development, children learn to control the sounds produced by their vocal tracts and to string sounds together. This period will give rise to the linguistic phase, whereby children begin to use words with consistent phonetic forms. The ages at which children meet the milestones proposed by Oller are approximate with overlap between the stages. As outlined by Oller, children's course to spoken language begins at birth with the Phonation Stage, which is characterized by the production of reflexive and vegetative sounds. This stage lasts through the first month of life and gives way to the Coo and Goo Stage (2–3 months). Vocalizations produced during this time are very similar to the adult form of the velar /k/ and /g/ and are paired with vowel-like sounds. During the Exploration and Expansion Stage (4–6 months), infants produce marginal babbling with fully resonated vowels. Vocal play is the highlight of this period, and children will produce significant variation in pitch and loudness of their utterances. Parents delight in the squeals, trills, and raspberries characteristic of this phase of development. The Canonical Babbling Stage occurs next with the emergence of reduplicated and variegated babbling. During reduplicated babbling, strings of very similar Consonant Vowel (CV) syllables are produced. Variegated babbling is a more complex feat, because infants produce different consonants and vowels in adjacent CV syllables. The Jargon Stage (10 months and older), characterized by variegated babbling with adult-like intonation, is the final phase before children transition to the production of first words (Oller, 1980).

During prelinguistic development, vowels dominate utterances with the earliest acquired consonants being the stops /t d k g p b/, the nasals /m, n/, the fricative /h/, and the glide /w/. Children's early syllable shapes will consist primarily of single V syllables, CV syllables, and CVCV forms. The transition from babbling to first words occurs around 9 to 18 months of age (Stoel-Gammon & Dunn, 1985). The initial precursor to first words are known as vocables, meaningless utterances that sound like true words, but are context specific and may be produced in conjunction with a consistent gesture. Following vocables are protowords, also known as phonetically consistent forms (PCFs) or invented words. These forms are not actual adult words but function as words for children and will be both phonetically and semantically consistent. Protowords are thought to serve as the link between babbling and adult-like speech. As children move toward the linguistic phase, there will be overlap in the use of protowords and "true words" in their communication attempts. True words have a consistent phonetic form and will be used consistently in a specific context. As children first attempt words, they will try words that contain phonemes already in their phonetic repertoire (Schwartz and Leonard, 1982).

The linguistic phase, a time of tremendous phonological development, begins around 12 months of age and consists of the child's first 50 words. This period is signaled by the rapid acquisition of new phonemes and sound patterns as children make strides toward adult-standard speech.

The development of consonant acquisition and phonological patterns appears to be largely universal, but there is significant variability in regard to specific ages for mastery as shown by research findings (Poole, 1934; Prather, Hendrick, & Kern, 1975; Templin, 1957; Grunwell, 1987). Although there is variation across studies, there is consensus that, in terms of development, children aquire certain categories of speech sounds before others. Nasals, stops, and glides are categories that are attained first and are followed by the acquisition of fricatives,

7 Steps of Phonological Acquisition		
Step	**Age**	**Stage**
1	1 year	Canonical babbling and vocables
2	$1\frac{1}{2}$ years	Recognizable words; CV structures; stops, nasals, glides
3	2 years	Final consonants, communication with words, "syllableness"
4	3 years	/s/ clusters, anterior-posterior contrasts, expansion of phonemic repertoire
5	4 years	Omissions rare, most "simplifications" suppressed, "adult-like" speech
6	5–6 years	Liquids /l/ (5 yrs) and /r/ (6 yrs), phonemic inventory stabilized
7	7 years	Sibilants and "th" perfected, "adult standard" speech

Source: Hodson (1997)

Fig. 3.2: Seven Steps of Phonological Acquisition

affricates, and lastly liquids. These categories of speech sound will be discussed in Chapter Six. Barbara Hodson (1997) proposed seven steps of phonological acquisition to assist speech-language pathologists (SLPs) in determining if a child is following typical phonological development.

The following graphs outline general ages of acquisition, according to findings of researchers, and highlight variability among the research conclusions.

Age of Phoneme Acquisition for Boys		
Age of Acquisition	**First Half of Year**	**Second Half of Year**
3	/p, b, m , n, w/ beginning /h/	/t, d, k/ beginning /f/
4	/g/	
5	beginning /j/	"tw" "kw" /v/ ending /f/
6	beginning /l/ and l-blends	
7	/ŋ, ð, s, z, ʃ, ʧ, ʤ/ "skw" "spl" s-blends ending /l/	
8	/θ/ r-blends "er" beginning /r/	
9	"spr" "thr" "skr" "str"	

(continued)

Age of Phoneme Acquisition for Girls		
Age of Acquisition	**First Half of Year**	**Second Half of Year**
3	/p, b, m , d, w/ beginning /h/	/g, k, n/ beginning /f/
4	/j, t/ "tw" "kw"	/θ/
5	beginning /l/	/v/ l-blends ending /f/
6	/ʤ, ʧ, θ, ʃ/ ending /l/	
7	/ŋ, s, z,/ "skw" "spl" s-blends	
8	r-blends "er" beginning /r/	
9	"spr" "thr" "skr" "str"	

Fig. 3.3: Age of Phoneme Acquisition

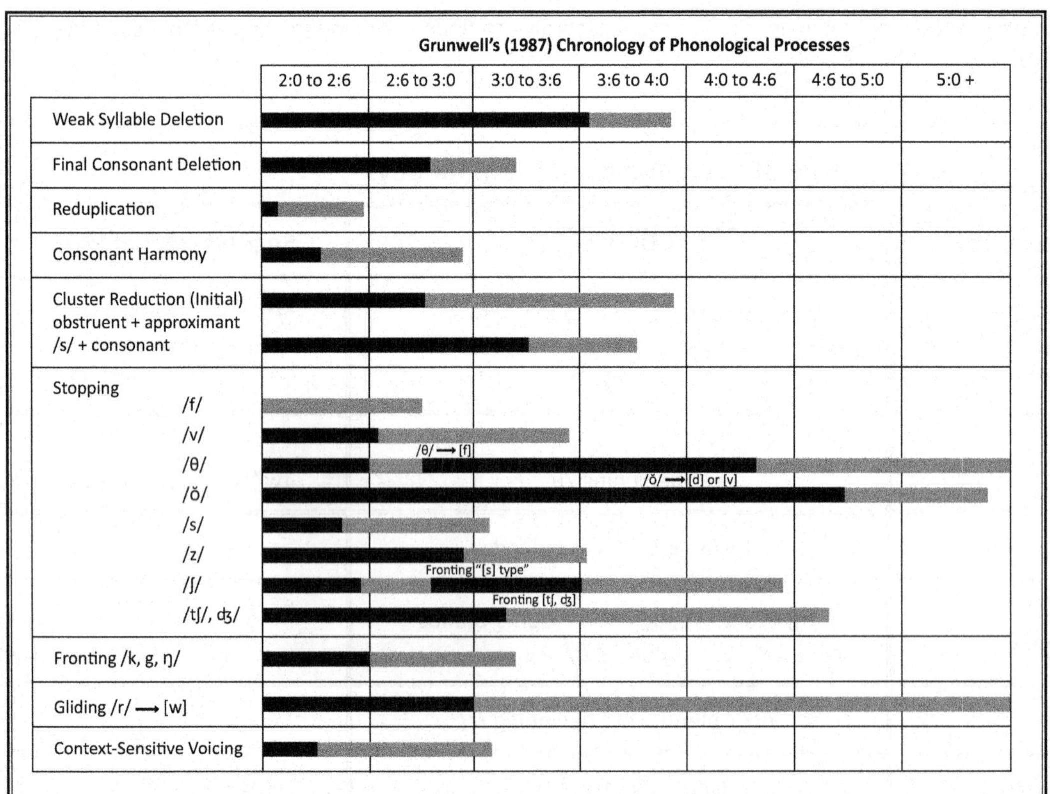

Fig. 3.4: Grunwell's (1987) Chronology of Phonological Processes

PHONOLOGICAL AWARENESS

Phonological awareness refers to children's ability to understand phonological rules to the extent that they can manipulate the sound structure of words (Robertson and Salter, 1997). Expressively, by age 4 to 5, children produce adult-like speech, but may still be developing the liquids, refining some sibilants and interdental sounds, and mastering consonant clusters and multisyllabic words on into the early elementary school years (Hodson, 1997). By age 7, children, from an expressive standpoint, generally have well-developed phonological systems. Receptively, during the early preschool years, children begin to understand that words are composed of individual sounds, and it is during this time that phonological awareness abilities emerge and continue to develop throughout the school age years. These skills include: manipulating the sound structure of a word, rhyming, segmenting words into their individual syllables and sounds components, sound blending, alliteration, identifying sounds within the word, and deleting sounds from words. Activities designed to facilitate phonological awareness help children think about the internal structure of words. Research has suggested that some children demonstrate phonological awareness as early as 2 to 3 years of age (Lonigan, Burgess, Anthony, & Barker, 1998), while others don't start to demonstrate these abilities until age 4 or 5 (Dodd & Gillon, 2001). These skills are vital to the acquisition of literacy, and children with expressive phonological disorders may be at risk for reading and writing difficulties (Hodson & Strattman, 2004).

The following are some common phonological awareness tasks.

Rhyming: Add a rhyming word to each example.

Orthographic	IPA
blue	/blu/
clue	/klu/
mitt	/mɪt/
pit	/pɪt/
cat	/kæt/

(*continued*)

hat	/hæt/
game	/gem/
name	/nem/
flew	/flu/
through	/θru/

Segmenting Words into Syllables and Sounds:

Orthographic Word	Syllables	IPA Word	IPA Sounds
cat	cat (1)	/kæt/	(3)
table	ta-ble (2)	/tebl̩/	(4)
banana	ba-na-na (3)	/bənænə/	(6)

reinforcement	re-in-force-ment (4)	/riɛnfɔrsmɛnt/	(12)
originated	o-ri-gi-nat-ed (5)	/ərɪʤənetɛd/	(10)

**this graph can be reversed to show syllables into words and sounds into words*

Recognition of Sounds at Beginning of Words

Orthographic	IPA
cat	/k/
cape	/k/
kind	/k/
crunch	/kr/
cog	/k/

Recognition of Sounds in Middle of Words

Orthographic	IPA
that	/æ/
ran	/æ/

(*continued*)

tan	/æ/
clan	/æ/
brand	/æ/

Recognition of Sounds at End of Words

Orthographic	IPA
jump	/mp/
blimp	/mp/
stamp	/mp/
nap	/p/
trap	/p/

THEORIES OF PHONOLOGICAL DEVELOPMENT

The field of speech-language pathology has benefited greatly from research in the area of linguistics, particularly in regard to our understanding of phonology and the ways in which children acquire speech sound systems. The following are discussions of several theories put forth to explain how sound systems organize to form phonological rules. Currently, no single theory adequately explains phonological development, nor is there a consensus among researchers on how speech acquisition occurs. However, these theories have contributed insights into how children become talkers, thereby furthering the field of speech-language pathology, both from assessment and from intervention standpoints.

Behavioral Theory

This explanation of speech acquisition is based on behaviorist theories of psychology proposed by Skinner (1953), Olmsted (1966), and Mower (1952) and is centered on the idea that children are directly conditioned by the environment and by the reinforcement of their verbal communication. The child's role is seen as passive; the development of speech sounds to communicate is the result of caregivers "shaping" the infant's babbling through contingent reinforcement. When the child produces sounds that match phonemes of the language spoken by the caregivers, the infant's utterance is reinforced. In addition to the selective reinforcement by adults in the environment, infants also begin to notice the similarities in the sounds they are producing and those provided by their caregivers. This theory emphasizes the role that babbling plays to advance meaningful speech, as well as the contributions of input and speech sound perception. Behavioral Theory is a key component to many speech sound interventions.

Distinctive Feature Theory

Roman Jakobson (1941, 1968) proposed a theory based on the assumption that speech sounds are composed of a set of indivisible "features" that represent acoustic and articulatory properties of sounds. These features are presented in a binary system in which the feature is either present (+) or absent (-). No two phonemes will share the same features; however, there are groups of speech sounds that share many features, and these are referred to as "natural phoneme classes."

This theory suggests that there is an innate and universal acquisition of "feature contrasts," rather than an attainment of individual speech sounds. Acquired feature contrasts follow a predictable pattern, beginning with sounds with maximal difference, such as consonants versus vowels sounds, oral versus nasal sounds, and anterior versus posterior sounds. This theory does not support a link from babbling to meaningful speech or recognize a rule-based nature of phonological systems. Furthermore, although some children do appear to acquire certain sound classes before others, a universal order of development is not seen across all children and lacks consistent research support.

Generative Phonology

This theory put forth by Chomsky and Halle (a student of Jakobson) in 1968 is an extension of the Distinctive Features Theory. Chomsky and Halle used distinctive features to describe phonological rules to explain the differences between the underlying representations (the hypothesized mental representations of words to which phonological rules apply) and surface forms (the actual sounds produced by the speech mechanism) of a word. Sounds, which share features, form natural sound classes. Speech sounds are characterized as either "marked" or "natural." Natural sounds are usually the earliest to develop, because they are easier for the child to produce. They are also more often represented in languages spoken throughout the world. Marked sounds, on the other hand, are more challenging to produce and occur less frequently in world languages. The nasal /m/ as in "mom" would be considered a natural sound, because it is early developing, relatively easy to produce, and represented in many languages. In contrast, the liquid /r/ would be considered marked, because it is later developing, difficult to produce, and is not represented in languages as often as other phonemes.

There are two levels of development proposed by this theory: surface level and deep level. The surface level is what is actually spoken by the child, while the deep level deals with the child's mental representation of language. The details of how phonemes are stored in the brain are called phonological representations. A child's knowledge of phonemes is placed on a continuum ranging from 1, complete knowledge of the sound, to 6, absence of the sound from the child's phonetic inventory.

Clinically, this theory has been useful in describing children's sound errors according to phonological rules; however, due to its abstract nature, the notion of phonological rules has been questioned.

Natural Phonology

Natural Phonology is a theory advanced by Stampe in 1969 to explain the common aspects of languages and the predictable manner in which children acquire sound systems, irrespective of the language that is being learned. Stampe theorized that, due to the limitations of their developing motor systems, children approximate adult speech by using innate and universal "natural" phonological processes that reflect the capability of their burgeoning motoric development. He proposed that these processes are innate, universal, and imperative to the developing talker in simplifying the production of sounds and sound sequences. Three broad classifications were identified: syllable structure processes, sound substitution processes, and assimilatory processes. As children mature, physical changes will also result in changes in their phonological systems. Stampe outlined three mechanisms by which these changes take place:

Limitation: Children gradually decrease the occurrences in which certain processes are used. For example, early in development, a child might delete all final consonants, but over time, might begin to use all possible final consonants except for stops.

Ordering: Children reorganize the application of individual processes so that some are no longer used in certain sequences.

Suppression: Children suppress processes to the extent that they are no longer used.

Stampe's Natural Phonology Theory gave rise to Clinical Phonology beginning in the 1970s. This theory has been useful to researchers in the clinical arena when developing therapeutic goals and assessing disorders.

Prosodic Theory

This theory advanced by Waterson (1970) proposes that the variability seen in the acquisition of speech across children is related to the uniqueness of a child's input. This theory considers the child an active learner who perceives whole words rather than segmental units; therefore, it is considered a "nonsegmental" theory. Instead of segmental units, the child picks up on prosodic features and the syllable structure of words for phonological development. Children will also begin to observe similarities among words that share common features, and as their perception increases, so will their production of words.

Cognitive Theories

Unlike Behavioral Theory, which saw infants as passive learners whose speech production was shaped by the environment, cognitive theories (e.g., Macken and Ferguson 1983) center on children as active learners who seek out their own phonological rules as they try to bridge the gap between sounds perceived in the environment and their own production of speech sounds. This theory focuses on the early stages of speech acquisition with children discovering the rules of language by developing and testing their own hypotheses about language structure. Accordingly, phonological rules are not seen as innate, because children actively develop their own strategies. This may account for individual variation in phonological acquisition seen among children.

Nonlinear Theories

Several nonlinear theories (e.g., Bernhardt and Stoel-Gammon, 1994) have advanced, each dealing with some aspect of sound segments, syllables, and words. These theories question the notion that a phoneme is composed of independent and unorganized features that may combine with one another without restrictions. The major underlying theme uniting nonlinear theories is that there is a hierarchical relationship among linguistic units that occur on different "tiers." Nonlinear theories also account for the effect that prosody has on speech production (Yavas, 1998). Clinically, nonlinear phonology has furthered our understanding of the production of multisyllabic words, and it has also contributed to the ways in which therapy is organized.

Metrical Phonology

This theory is concerned with prosodic features, particularly stress. The hierarchical relationship of "syllables," "feet," and "segments" is outlined and presented in tiers. Syllables are made up of the onset, rime, and coda. The onset includes the consonant, either singleton or blend, that comes before the vowel. The vowel serves as the nucleus of the syllable, and the rime includes the vowel and any consonants that follow it. Finally, the coda contains the consonants that follow the nucleus. Stressed syllables and one or more unstressed syllables comprise a "foot." When stress is varied across syllables, speech rhythm results.

Feature Geometry

As with metrical phonology, feature geometry uses tiers to present the relationship of features within segments. Some features will be dominant, while others will combine more readily with particular features. A "node" would be considered a dominant feature and, thus, higher in the hierarchy. Feature spreading is a concept similar to assimilation and accounts for how some features influence the production of other features.

CONCLUSION

Although it is widely accepted that children come into our world hardwired to communicate, there is little consensus among researchers regarding how spoken language develops. Research has suggested, however, a somewhat predictable order of acquisition for sound development. As far as phonology is concerned, some theories have been proposed that represent the phoneme as a bundle of independent features that can combine freely, while other theories emphasize the hierarchical relationship among segmental units. Research in the area of speech acquisition and development and phonological awareness has advanced the field of speech-language pathology and informed clinical practice.

IMAGE CREDITS

- Fig 3.1: R.D. Kent and A.D. Murray, "Comparison of Infant and Adult Oral Structures," Journal of Acoustical Society of America, vol. 72, pp. 353. Copyright © 1982 by AIP Publishing LLC. Reprinted with permission.
- Fig 3.2: Barbara Hodson and Mary Louis Edwards, "7 Steps of Phonological Acquisition," Perspectives in Applied Phonology. Copyright © 1997 by PRO-ED, Inc.
- Fig 3.4: Pamela Grunwell, "Chronology of Phonological Processes," Clinical Phonology, p. 183. Copyright © 1981 by Croom Helm.

CHAPTER

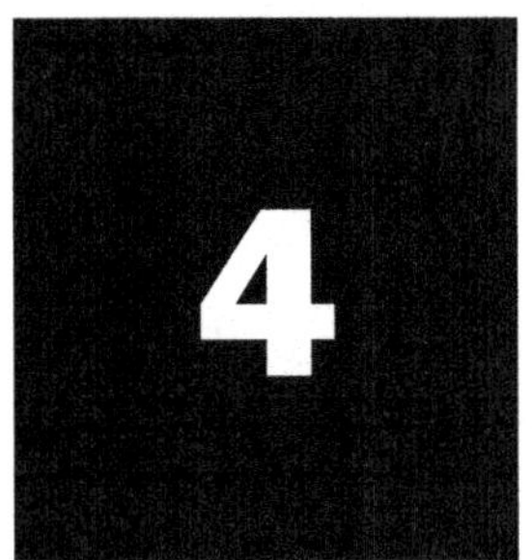

As was discussed in Chapter 2, vocal fold vibration provides a sound source, making the production of vowels possible. Vowels are crucial to speech, because they provide power to our words. Try speaking using only consonant speech sounds, and the importance of vowels as the power source to speech will become apparent. Vowels form the nucleus of the syllables that comprise words. A syllable must contain a vowel (monophthong or diphthong), which may be surrounded by one or more consonants.

The production of different vowels is the result of adjusting the size and shape of the vocal tract, which can be thought of like a tube formed by the mouth and throat (Ladefoged, 2005). When the vocal folds open and close, pulses of air are released, which cause the air in the vocal tract to be set into motion, producing vibrations. The vocal tract has a complex shape that is capable of producing different acoustic properties or **resonances** (Ladefoged, 2005). These resonances can be thought of as "bands of concentrated energy" and are referred to as **formants.** Although there are an endless number of formants, only the first two or three are needed in identifying vowels, and they are used to characterize resonant consonants (Edwards, 2003). Tongue height, tongue advancement, and lip shape will produce a formant structure unique to each vowel (Chomsky & Halle, 1968).

THE ENGLISH VOWEL SYSTEM

When you think of vowels, you may recall the familiar "a, e, i, o, u, and sometimes y" from primary school. The English vowel system, however, is much more complex. Most English vowels are **monophthongs,** or "pure vowels," which have a single and consistent sound quality (Van Riper & Smith, 1979). **Diphthongs** are vowels that have a characteristic that changes during production, resulting in a complex and dynamic sound quality (Ladefoged, 2005). During production, there is a gradually shifting articulation, which consists of an **ong-lide** (the position of the articulators at the beginning of one vowel) and an **off-glide** (the position of the articulators at the end of another vowel). Most often, the off-glide has a higher tongue position than the on-glide.

Vowels are characterized by the following:

1. Shaping of the oral cavity:

Every vowel will have a characteristic vocal tract shape that is determined by how the tongue, jaw, and lips are positioned.

(a) **Tongue height** is a description of the vertical position of the tongue body. The distance between the tongue and the hard palate ranges from high to low height. The following words contain vowels ranging from high to low tongue height: meet→mit→mate→met→mat.

(b) **Tongue position (or advancement)** is a description of the positioning of the tongue body ranging from front to back of the mouth. The following words contain vowels proceeding from front to back: meet→mutt→moot.

(c) **Tenseness versus laxness** is a description of the degree of tension of vocal musculature (particularly the tongue) during production. Tense vowels are longer in duration; lax vowels have a shorter duration, and the degree of muscular effort is less extensive (Shriberg & Kent, 1995). The following two words are produced with a tense and lax vowel, respectively: meet→mit.

(d) **Jaw position** is a description of the openness of the mandible (jaw). There are four mandible positions during vowel production that influence vowel height (House, 1998).

- *Open*—This position is similar to your doctor's directions to, "Open up and say *ahhhh.*" The "*ahhhh*" /ɑ/ is actually a back vowel with the tongue in the lowest vertical position and the jaw open. Because the jaw supports the tongue, the tongue will follow the jaw's direction during the production of vowels. When the jaw is completely open, the tongue will rest on the floor of the mouth. Say "*Ahhhh*" /ɑ/ to get a feel for the tongue when the jaw is in the open position.
- *Mid-open*—The mandible is slightly elevated, but not completely open placing the tongue somewhat raised from the floor of the mouth. Say "*Uh,*" /ʌ/ as in the word *up*, to get a feel for the tongue when the jaw is in the mid-open position.
- *Mid-closed*—For this position, the jaw is almost closed, but the back teeth do not touch. The tongue is halfway between the floor of the mouth and the palates (hard and soft). Say *"Oh"* /o/ as in the word *open* to get a feel for the tongue when the jaw is in the mid-closed position.
- *Closed*—The jaw is in an elevated position, thereby causing the tongue to be in contact with the sides of the alveolar ridge. Say *"Eee"* /i/ as in the word *eat* to get a feel for the tongue when the jaw is in the closed position.

(e) **Lip configuration** is a description of the degree of lip rounding, which will lengthen the vocal tract, thereby influencing the acoustic characteristics of certain vowels. The lips can be either rounded or unrounded (spread). The following two words are produced with lips rounded and unrounded, respectively: moot→meet.

2. Vocal fold vibration:

The vocal folds are adducted for voicing, because all vowels are voiced.

3. Velopharyngeal closure:

All vowels are oral speech sounds and will be produced with the velopharyngeal port closed, allowing the voiced airstream to be directed out of the mouth.

FRONT	CENTRAL	BACK	
/i/		/u/	HIGH
/ɪ/		/ʊ/	HIGH-MID
/e/	/ɝ/ /ə/ /ɚ/	/o/	MID
/ɛ/		/ɔ/	LOW-MID
/æ/		/ɑ/	LOW

Fig. 4.1 Quad

FRONT	CENTRAL	BACK	
			HIGH
			HIGH-MID
			MID
			LOW-MID
			LOW

Fig. 4.2 QuadBlank

THE VOWEL QUADRILATERAL

The Vowel Quadrilateral is a schematic of how the different vowel sounds are displayed on the tongue.

To illustrate the many differences between orthographic and phonetic representation of vowels, the common and less common spellings for each vowel presented in this text will be shown, starting with the most frequently used spellings.

Several exercises are presented in this chapter to assist in transcribing the 14 monophthongs, 4 diphthongs, 5 rhotic diphthongs, and 2 rhotic triphthongs in the English vowel system using the International Phonetic Alphabet (IPA). IPA symbols for consonants that are familiar to you will be used in these exercises. The following is a guide to help when completing the exercises.

p as in *pup* =	/p /	*f* as in *food* =	/f/
b as in *boy* =	/b/	*v* as in *vent* =	/v/
t as in *tea* =	/t/	*h* as in *hot* =	/h/
d as in *dog* =	/d/	*n* as in *no* =	/n/
k as in *king* =	/k/	*m* as in *mom* =	/m/
g as in *gift* =	/g/	*r* as in *run* =	/r/
s as *say* =	/s/	*l* as in *lake* =	/l/
z as in *zoo* =	/z/	*w* as in *wait* =	/w/

Before you begin transcribing:

When transcribing someone's speech, it is imperative that you transcribe the person's words as *they* produced them, not as you would say them. We all say words a little differently. Think of the old song with the familiar phrase, "You say *toemay-toe*, I say *tuh-mah-toe*." It doesn't matter if you say *toemay-toe* /tometo/, if you are transcribing the speech of a person who says *tuh-mah-toe* /təmɑto/, then you transcribe /təmɑto/ not /tometo/. This will be an extremely difficult task at first. Practice transcribing the speech of someone from a different part of the country who speaks a slightly different dialect than that spoken by your speech community. This will help you experience the vowel variations that different speakers use.

Remember the way words are spelled and the way they are pronounced are, for the most part, poorly related to each other. For example, words are often spelled using "silent" letters, e.g., *come* (the e at the end is silent), or they are spelled using double letters to indicate one speech sound, e.g., *rabbit* (the double bb in the middle represents just one sound); these words would be transcribed /kʌm/ and /ræbɪt/, respectively. As much as it is possible, try to "forget" how the words you are transcribing are spelled and concentrate on how they sound.

Also, keep in mind that there are no capitalization and punctuation rules in phonetic transcription. The symbols representing different speech sounds will not change regardless of how the words are being used to convey messages. It will be difficult at first not to capitalize proper nouns and the first word of a sentence, but as with all things, practice will help you become more proficient at phonetic transciption.

Another unique aspect of phonetic transcription is that homophones will have a consistent transcription. Homophones are words that sound the same, but have different meanings and are spelled differently. *Blue* and blew are homophones, and both would be transcribed /blu/ irrespective of how they are being used in a sentence.

When transcribing, you can never practice too much! Phonetic transcription is a difficult skill that requires hours upon hours of practice for you to become proficient. The key to becoming a skilled transcriber is to practice, practice, practice, and then, practice some more.

The next section of this chapter will introduce the 14 monophthongs, 4 diphthongs, 5 rhotic diphthongs, and 2 rhotic triphthongs commonly used in English. Each section will include practice exercises designed to help you become a better transcriber. For the practice items, enclose all IPA symbols within virgules / /.

Monophthongs

The Front Vowels

As the name implies, the front vowels are produced with the tongue toward the front of the mouth. The front portion of the tongue is the most involved in creating each of the five front vowels: /i ɪ e ɛ æ/.

The following is the sequence for producing the **front** vowels:

1. Vocal folds are adducted (closed) so that vocal fold vibration occurs, because all vowels are voiced.
2. The velum touches the back of throat so that velopharyngeal closure occurs, ensuring the vibrated air is directed out the mouth, because all vowels are oral speech sounds.
3. The tongue is positioned toward the **front** of the mouth.
4. The tongue will be elevated to different heights depending on which **front** vowel is being produced.

High:	/i/
Mid-High:	/ɪ/
Mid:	/e/
Mid-Low:	/ɛ/
Low:	/æ/

5. The tongue will be tense or lax depending on which **front** vowel is being produced.

Tense:	/i / and /e/
Lax:	/ɪ/, /ɛ/, and /æ/

6. The lips are unrounded for all of the **front** vowels.
7. The jaw will vary according to the degree it is opened.

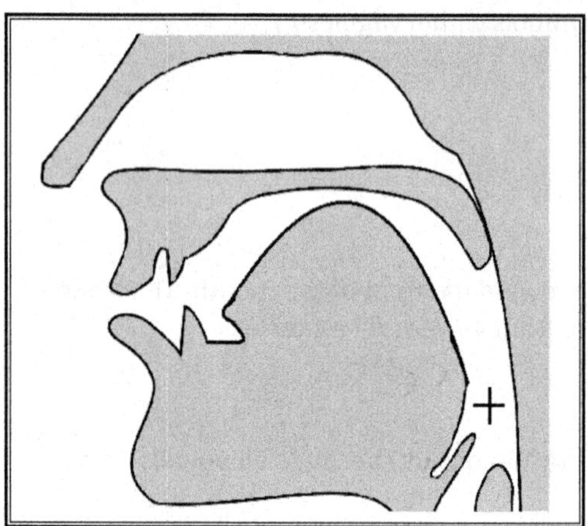

Fig. 4.3: i

/i/: Keyword *Bee*/bi/

Tongue height: High

Tongue position: Front

Degree of tongue tension: Tense

Degree of lip rounding: Unrounded

Common spellings beginning with the most commonly used (Hanna et al., 1966):

e:	We
ee:	Bee
ea:	Tea
i-e:	Believe
ei:	Receive
eo:	People
ey:	Key

Exercise 4.1 Transcribe the following words containing /i/. Remember that all consonants in this exercise are the same as orthography:

1. beam	/bim/	6. Keen	/Kin/
2. dean	/din/	7. lean	/lin/
3. ease	/iz/	8. heat	/hit/
4. free	/fri/	9. peace	/pis/
5. glee	/gli/	10. greet	/grit/

Exercise 4.2 Identify the following words:

1. /fli/	flee	6. /lig/	league
2. /drim/	dream	7. /mik/	meek
3. /krip/	creep	8. /did/	deed
4. /bist/	beast	9. /grin/	green
5. /lif/	leaf	10. /hip/	heap

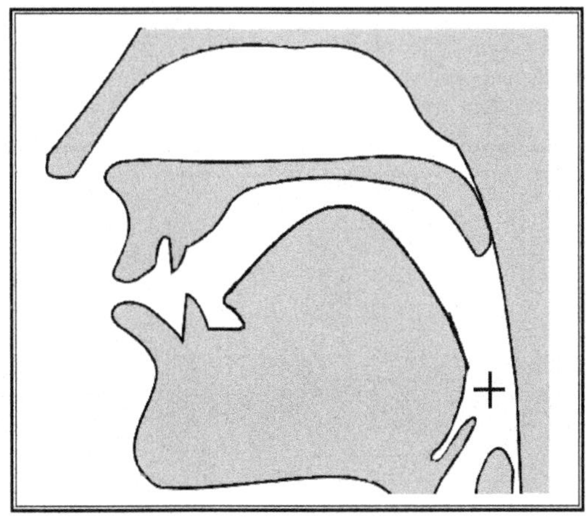

Fig. 4.4: /I/

/ɪ/ Keyword: *Bit* /bɪt/

Tongue height: Mid-High

Tongue position: Front

Degree of tongue tension: Lax

Degree of lip rounding: Unrounded

Common spellings beginning with the most commonly used (Hanna et al., 1966):

i:	Wit
y:	Hymn
e:	Pretty
a-e:	Image
ei:	Receive
o:	Lemon
ui:	Build

Exercise 4.3 Transcribe the following words containing /ɪ/. Remember that all consonants in this exercise are the same as orthography:

1. bid	/bɪd/	6. him	/hɪm/
2. tin	/tɪn/	7. lip	/lɪp/
3. pig	/pɪg/	8. kid	/kɪd/
4. dim	/dɪm/	9. fig	/fɪg/
5. lid	/lɪd/	10. fin	/fɪn/

Exercise 4.4 Identify the following words:

1. /bɪg/	big	6. /dɪd/	did
2. /pɪn/	pin	7. /fɪn/	fin
3. /tɪp/	tip	8. /lɪd/	lid
4. /hɪt/	hit	9. /grɪn/	grin
5. /dɪg/	dig	10. /hɪp/	hip

Exercise 4.5 Differentiate /i/ and /ɪ/by circling the vowel in each word:

evil	/i/	/ɪ/	lid	/i/	/ɪ/
hymn	/i/	/ɪ/	seam	/i/	/ɪ/
gym	/i/	/ɪ/	these	/i/	/ɪ/
ski	/i/	/ɪ/	give	/i/	/ɪ/
built	/i/	/ɪ/	eve	/i/	/ɪ/
tea	/i/	/ɪ/	list	/i/	/ɪ/
seat	/i/	/ɪ/	sieve	/i/	/ɪ/
ship	/i/	/ɪ/	feast	/i/	/ɪ/
seek	/i/	/ɪ/	skip	/i/	/ɪ/
rich	/i/	/ɪ/	risk	/i/	/ɪ/

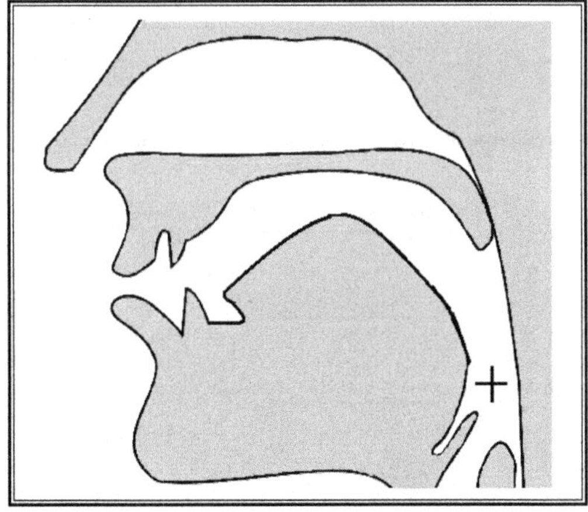

Fig. 4.5: e

/e/ Keyword: *Ate* /et/

Tongue height: Mid

Tongue position: Front

Degree of tongue tension: Tense

Degree of lip rounding: Unrounded

Common spellings beginning with the most commonly used (Hanna et al., 1966):

a: Table

a-e: Mate

(*Continued*)

ai:	Pain
ea:	Break
ay:	Day

Exercise 4.6 Transcribe the following words containing /e/. Remember that all consonants in this exercise are the same as orthography:

1. bait	/bet/	6. gain	/gen/
2. dane	/den/	7. braid	/bred/
3. train	/tren/	8. hay	/he/
4. brain	/bren/	9. plate	/plet/
5. fain	/fen/	10. aim	/em/

Exercise 4.7 Identify the following words:

1. /ren/	rain	6. /wet/	wait
2. /dren/	drain	7. /fes/	face
3. /plen/	plain	8. /pest/	paste
4. /le/	lay	9. /gren/	grain
5./wev/	wave	10. /greps/	grapes

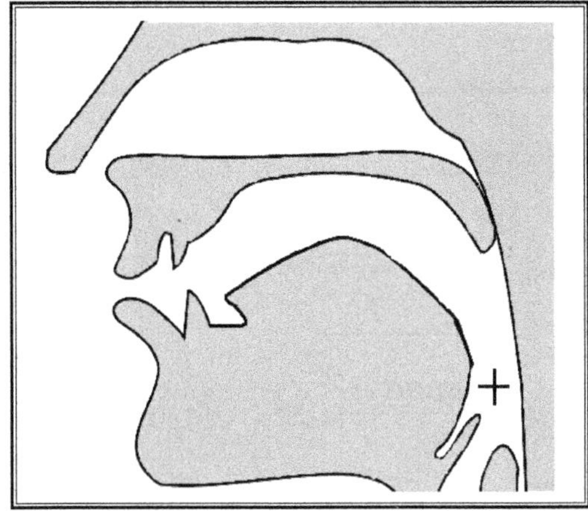

Fig. 4.6: 3

/ɛ/ Keyword: *Pet* /pɛt/

Tongue height: Mid-Low

Tongue position: Front

Degree of tongue tension: Lax

Degree of lip rounding: Unrounded

Common spellings beginning with the most commonly used (Hanna et al., 1966):

e:	Pen
a:	Any
ai:	Again
ea:	Meant
ei:	Heifer
ie:	Friend
ue:	Guest

Exercise 4.8 Transcribe the following words containing /ɛ/. Remember that all consonants in this exercise are the same as orthography:

1. beg	/bɛg/	6. desk	/dɛsk/
2. hen	/hɛn/	7. pest	/pɛst/
3. egg	/ɛg/	8. head	/hɛd/
4. wept	/wɛpt/	9. guest	/gɛst/
5. leg	/lɛg/	10. guess	/gɛs/

Exercise 4.9 Identify the following words:

1. /ɛlf/	elf	6. /lɛft/	left
2. /frɛnd/	friend	7. /ɛnd/	end
3. /dɛt/	debt	8. /dɛd/	dead
4. /nɛlt/	knelt	9. /pɛn/	pen
5. /pɛg/	peg	10. /stɛpt/	stepped

Exercise 4.10 Differentiate /ɛ/ and /ɪ/ in minimal pairs by circling the vowel in each word:`

1.	wet	(/ɛ/)	/ɪ/	wit	/ɛ/	(/ɪ/)
2.	ten	(/ɛ/)	/ɪ/	tin	/ɛ/	(/ɪ/)
3.	beg	(/ɛ/)	/ɪ/	big	/ɛ/	(/ɪ/)
4.	mitt	/ɛ/	(/ɪ/)	met	(/ɛ/)	/ɪ/
5.	bed	(/ɛ/)	/ɪ/	bid	/ɛ/	(/ɪ/)
6.	set	(/ɛ/)	/ɪ/	sit	/ɛ/	(/ɪ/)
7.	net	(/ɛ/)	/ɪ/	knit	/ɛ/	(/ɪ/)
8.	bit	/ɛ/	(/ɪ/)	bet	(/ɛ/)	/ɪ/
9.	lit	/ɛ/	(/ɪ/)	let	(/ɛ/)	/ɪ/
10.	den	(/ɛ/)	/ɪ/	din	/ɛ/	(/ɪ/)

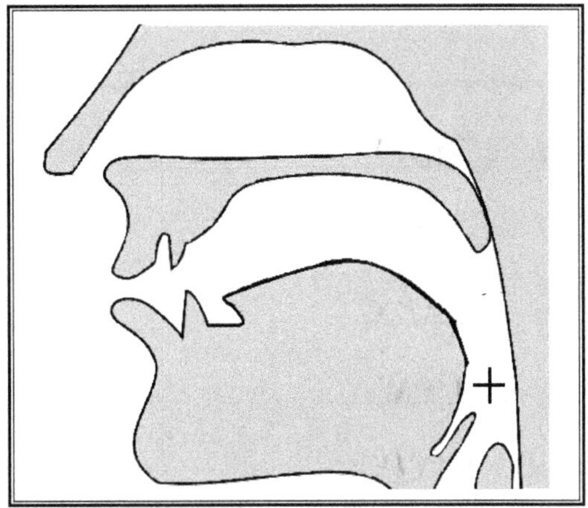

Fig. 4.7: ae

/æ/ Keywords: *Cat* /kæt/

Tongue height: Low

Tongue position: Front

Degree of tongue tension: Lax

Degree of lip rounding: Unrounded

Common spellings beginning with the most commonly used (Hanna et al., 1966):

a: Fat

au: Aunt

ai: Plaid

Exercise 4.11 Transcribe the following words containing /æ/. Remember that all consonants in this exercise are the same as orthography:

1. ask	/aesk/	6. gas	/gaes/
2. zap	/zaep/	7. bag	/baeg/
3. hat	/haet/	8. dab	/daeb/
4. sad	/saed/	9. map	/maep/
5. fat	/faet/	10. lab	/laeb/

Exercise 4.12 Identify the following words:

1. /bæs/	bass	6. /glæd/	glad
2. /æt/	at	7. /mæs/	mass
3. /læf/	laugh	8. /læst/	last
4. /kæf/	calf	9. /snæp/	snap
5./hæz/	has	10. /hæv/	have

Exercise 4.13 Transcribe the front vowels in the following words:

1. that	ae	15. chief	i
2. mate	e	16. his	I
3. jet	ɛ	17. tease	i
4. meet	i	18. rinse	I
5. nap	ae	19. knelt	ɛ
6. ray	e	20. lean	i
7. pat	ae	21. each	i
8. head	ɛ	22. mat	ae
9. pin	I	23. big	I
10. beach	i	24. age	e
11. day	e	25. gaze	e
12. beige	e	26. preach	i
13. peach	i	27. late	e
14. pain	e	28. rate	e

29. pet	ɛ	35. bat	æ
30. feed	i	36. black	æ
31. debt	ɛ	37. heave	i
32. leap	i	38. swim	ɪ
33. bait	e	39. speck	ɛ
34. date	e	40. lain	e

The Back Vowels

The back vowels differ from the front vowels in that the tongue is situated toward the back of the mouth, and it is the back portion of the tongue that is primarily engaged in their production. The back vowels are: /u ʊ o ɔ ɑ/.

The following is the sequence for producing the **back** vowels:

1. Vocal folds are adducted (closed) so that vocal fold vibration occurs, because all vowels are voiced.
2. The velum touches the back of throat so that velopharyngeal closure occurs, ensuring that the vibrated air is directed out the mouth, because all vowels are oral speech sounds.
3. The tongue is positioned toward the **back** of the mouth.
4. The tongue will be elevated to different heights depending on which **back** vowel is being produced.

High:	/u/
Mid-High:	/ʊ/
Mid:	/o/
Mid-Low:	/ɔ/
Low:	/ɑ/

5. The tongue will be tense or lax depending on which **back** vowel is being produced.

Tense:	/u/, /o/, /ɔ/, and /ɑ/
Lax:	/ʊ/

6. The lips will be rounded or unrounded. The back vowels /u ʊ o ɔ/ are rounded, /ɑ/ is unrounded.
7. The jaw will vary according the degree it is opened.

The influence of tongue depth can be realized by repeating the contrasting front vowel sound [i], heard in eat, and the back vowel [u], heard in ooze. Try each of the following front/back contrasts.

[i] eat	→	[u] ooze
[I] itch	→	[ʊ] book
[e] phonate	→	[o] robot
[ɛ] Ed	→	[ɔ] awful
[æ] ask	→	[ɑ] spa

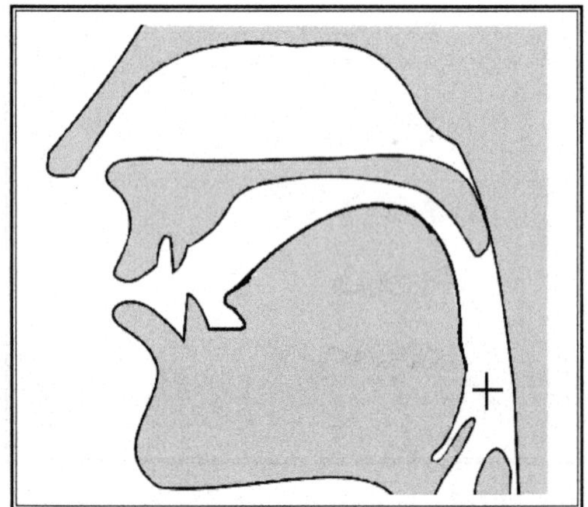

Fig. 4.8: u

/u/ Keyword: *Too* /tu/

Tongue height: High

Tongue position: Back

Degree of tongue tension: Tense

Degree of lip rounding: Rounded

Common spellings beginning with the most commonly used (Hanna et al., 1966):

oo:	Hoot
u:	Truly
u-e:	Rude
o:	To
oe:	Canoe

Exercise 4.14 Transcribe the following words containing /u/. Remember that all consonants in this exercise are the same as orthography:

1. moo	/mu/	6. two	/tu/
2. flute	/flut/	7. zoo	/zu/
3. prune	/prun/	8. tune	/tun/
4. blew	/blu/	9. spoon	/spun/
5. sue	/su/	10. plume	/plum/

Exercise 4.15 Identify the following words:

1. /flu/	flu	6. /gus/	goose
2. /dru/	drew	7. /sut/	suit
3. /muv/	move	8. /gru/	grew
4. /but/	boot	9. /grum/	groom
5. /brum/	broom	10. /hu/	who

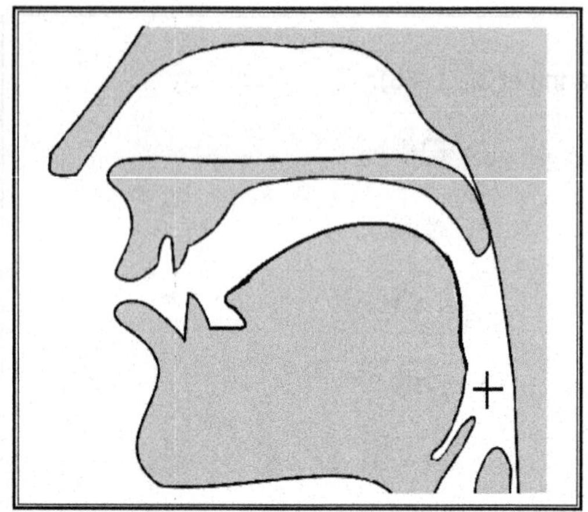

Fig. 4.9: oo

/ʊ/ Keyword: *H<u>oo</u>k* /hʊk/

Tongue height: Mid-High

Tongue position: Back

Degree of tongue tension: Lax

Degree of lip rounding: Rounded

Common spellings beginning with the most commonly used (Hanna et al., 1966):

u:	Sugar
oo:	Hook
ou:	Would

Exercise 4.16 Transcribe the following words containing /ʊ/. Remember that all consonants in this exercise are the same as orthography:

1. book /bʊk/
2. look /lʊk/
3. good /gʊd/
4. wood /wʊd/
5. cook /kʊk/
6. soot /sʊt/
7. foot /fʊt/
8. wool /wʊl/
9. put /pʊt/
10. wolf /wʊlf/

Exercise 4.17 Identify the following words:

1. /pʊl/	pull	6. /krʊk/	crook
2. /kʊd/	could	7. /tʊk/	took
3. /bʊks/	books	8. /brʊk/	brook
4. /wʊdz/	woods	9. /fʊt/	foot
5. /lʊkt/	looked	10. /hʊd/	hood

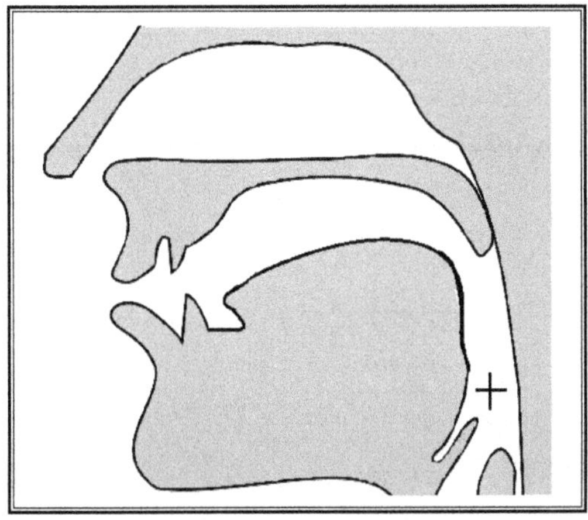

Fig. 4.10: o

/o/ Keyword: *b<u>oa</u>t* /bot/

Tongue height: Mid

Tongue position: Back

Degree of tongue tension: Tense

Degree of lip rounding: Rounded

Common spellings beginning with the most commonly used (Hanna et al., 1966):

o: <u>O</u>bey

o-e: T<u>o</u>t<u>e</u>

oa: B<u>oa</u>t

ew: S<u>ew</u>

ow: Sn<u>ow</u>

oe: T<u>oe</u>

Exercise 4.18 Transcribe the following words containing /o/. Remember that all consonants in this exercise are the same as orthography:

1. toad	/tod/	6. told	/told/
2. bone	/bon/	7. sold	/sold/
3. rode	/rod/	8. row	/ro/
4. beau	/bo/	9. slow	/slo/
5. post	/post/	10. mode	/mod/

Exercise 4.19 Identify the following words:

1. /flo/	flow	6. /logo/	logo
2. /kro/	crow	7. /kom/	comb
3. /bo/	beau	8. /dop/	dope
4. /bost/	boast	9. /gro/	grow
5. /lon/	loan	10. /hop/	hope

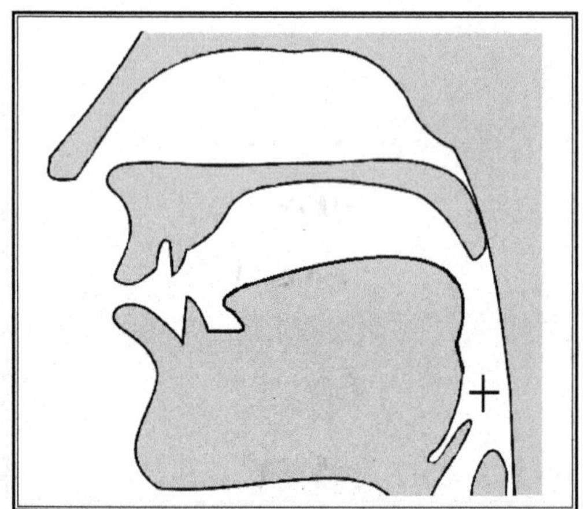

Fig. 4.11: aw

/ɔ/ Keyword: *saw* /sɔ/

Tongue height: Mid-Low

Tongue position: Back

Degree of tongue tension: Lax

Degree of lip rounding: Rounded

Common spellings beginning with the most commonly used (Hanna et al., 1966):

o:	Lost
a:	All
au:	Fault
aw:	Pawn
augh:	Caught
hau:	Exhaust
ough:	Fought

Exercise 4.20 Transcribe the following words containing /ɔ/. Remember that all consonants in this exercise are the same as orthography:

1. law	/lɔ/	6. off	/ɔf/
2. flaw	/flɔ/	7. raw	/rɔ/
3. spawn	/spɔn/	8. paw	/pɔ/
4. drawn	/drɔn/	9. caught	/kɔt/
5. scrawl	/skrɔl/	10. salt	/sɔlt/

Exercise 4.21 Identify the following words:

1. /sɔ/	saw	6. /lɔ/	law
2. /lɔn/	lawn	7. /kɔzd/	caused
3. /krɔl/	crawl	8. /frɔd/	fraud
4. /pɔn/	pawn	9. /fɔlt/	fault
5. /skɔld/	scald	10. /hɔnt/	haunt

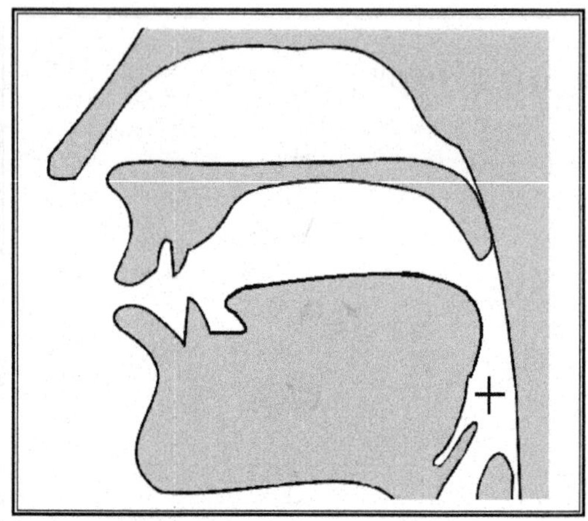
Fig. 4.12: ah

/ɑ/ Keyword: *Dog* /dɑg/

Tongue height: Low

Tongue position: Back

Degree of tongue tension: Lax

Degree of lip rounding: Unrounded

Common spellings beginning with the most commonly used (Hanna et al., 1966):

o:	Top
aa:	Bazaar
ua:	Guard
e:	Sergeant
ea:	Hearth
ho:	Honest

Exercise 4.22 Transcribe the following words containing /ɑ/. Remember that all consonants in this exercise are the same as orthography:

1. hot	/hat/	6. blot	/blat/
2. trot	/trat/	7. slot	/slat/
3. lot	/lat/	8. pot	/pat/
4. knot	/nat/	9. dot	/dat/
5. got	/gat/	10. swap	/swap/

Exercise 4.23 Identify the following words:

1. /taps /	tops	6. /drap /	drop
2. /slab /	slob	7. /baks /	box
3. /klak /	clock	8. /pap/	pop
4. /faks /	fox	9. /mam /	mom
5./ naks /	knocks	10. /spa/	spa

Exercise 4.24 Differentiating /ɔ/ and /ɑ/ in minimal pairs. Circle the vowel in each word:

1. hawk	/ɔ/ [circled]	/ɑ/	hock	/ɔ/	/ɑ/ [circled]
2. Don	/ɔ/	/ɑ/ [circled]	dawn	/ɔ/ [circled]	/ɑ/
3. odd	/ɔ/	/ɑ/ [circled]	awed	/ɔ/ [circled]	/ɑ/
4. raw	/ɔ/ [circled]	/ɑ/	rah	/ɔ/	/ɑ/ [circled]
5. cot	/ɔ/	/ɑ/ [circled]	caught	/ɔ/ [circled]	/ɑ/
6. sought	/ɔ/ [circled]	/ɑ/	sot	/ɔ/	/ɑ/ [circled]

Exercise 4.25 Transcribe the back vowels in the following words:

1. ooze	/u/	6. took	/ʊ/
2. caught	/ɔ/	7. boat	/o/
3. dog	/ɑ/	8. cook	/ʊ/
4. hope	/o/	9. grew	/u/
5. nope	/o/	10. soup	/u/

(Continued)

11. vote	/o/	26. hot	/ɑ/
12. brook	/ʊ/	27. all	/ɔ/
13. put	/ʊ/	28. pull	/ʊ/
14. draw	/ɔ/	29. snooze	/u/
15. true	/u/	30. shook	/ʊ/
16. rope	/o/	31. foot	/ʊ/
17. straw	/ɔ/	32. tube	/u/
18. book	/ʊ/	33. pause	/ɔ/
19. pop	/ɑ/	34. hook	/ʊ/
20. flute	/u/	35. drop	/ɑ/
21. cot	/ɑ/	36. rose	/o/
22. law	/ɔ/	37. group	/u/
23. fought	/ɔ/	38. scald	/ɔ/
24. toe	/o/	39. spot	/ɑ/
25. shoot	/u/	40. clue	/u/

Exercise 4.26 Transcribe the following words, which contain front and back vowels:

	Front		Back
1. bee	/bi/	boo	/bu/
2. pit	/pɪt/	put	/pʊt/
3. came	/kem/	comb	/kom/
4. pen	/pɛn/	pawn	/pɔn/

5. pat	/pæt/	pot	/pɑt/
6. key	/ki/	coo	/ku/
7. fit	/fɪt/	foot	/fʊt/
8. gate	/get/	goat	/got/
9. heck	/hɛk/	hawk	/hɔk/
10. slab	/slæb/	slob	/slɑb/

Central Vowels

The central vowels are produced with the tongue in the center of the mouth in a neutral position. Stress is vital to their description (Shriberg & Kent 1995). Different types of stress will be covered in detail in Chapter 5. The /ɝ/ and/ɚ/ are **rhotic** vowels, i.e., they have *r*-coloring. The unstressed non-rhotic central vowel /ə/ is referred to as the **schwa**, and the unstressed rhotic central vowel /ɚ/ is called the **schwar**.

The following is the sequence for producing the central vowels:

1. Vocal folds are adducted (closed) so that vocal fold vibration occurs, because all vowels are voiced.
2. The velum touches the back of throat so that velopharyngeal closure occurs, ensuring that the vibrated air is directed out of the mouth, because all vowels are oral speech sounds.
3. The tongue is positioned in a "neutral" position in the center of the mouth with very little variation in tongue position for the four vowels. The /ʌ/ and /ə/ tend to be made with a somewhat lower tongue position than /ɝ/ and /ɚ/, with /ʌ/ being made with the tongue in the back central portion of the tongue.
4. The tongue will be tense or lax depending on which central vowel is being produced.

Tense:	/ɝ/
Lax:	/ʌ/ /ə/ /ɚ/

5. The lips will be rounded or spread. The two rhotic central vowels /ɝ/ and /ɚ/ are produced with rounded lips.

As suggested by Shriberg & Kent (1995), stress is vital to the description of central vowels. For example, in the word burglar, there are two r-controlled central vowel sounds; the first syllable is stressed, and the second is unstressed: /ˈbɝglɚ/. It is the syllable stress that determines which central vowel is used. The [ˈ] symbol is used to indicate the primary stressed syllable.

Determining which central vowel to use can be a tough task for students. Monosyllabic words will always require the stressed versions /ʌ/ and /ɝ/. For example, *pun* and *curd* are monosyllabic words and are transcribed: /pʌn/ and /kɝd/. For words containing a central vowel with more than one syllable, if the syllable is unstressed, the central vowels /ə/ and /ɚ/ are used, and if the syllable is stressed, the stressed versions are used /ʌ/ and /ɝ/.

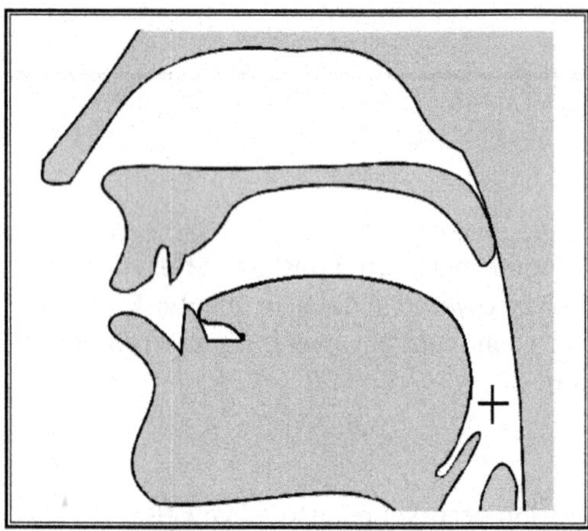

Fig. 4.13: (carrot)

/ʌ/ Keyword: *C<u>u</u>t* /kʌt/

Tongue height: Mid

Tongue position: Central

Degree of tongue tension: Lax

Degree of lip rounding: Unrounded

Common spellings beginning with the most commonly used (Hanna et al., 1966):

u:	Mutt
o:	Won
oe:	Does
ou:	Rough
oo:	Flood

Exercise 4.27 Transcribe the following words containing /ʌ/. Remember that all consonants in this exercise are the same as orthography:

1. bum	/bʌm/	6. mug	/mʌg/
2. dun	/dʌn/	7. sub	/sʌb/
3. cut	/kʌt/	8. hut	/hʌt/
4. bug	/bʌg/	9. dug	/dʌg/
5. gun	/gʌn/	10. bus	/bʌs/

Exercise 4.28 Read the phonetic symbols to identify the following words:

1. /flʌd/	flood	6. /lʌg/	lug
2. /drʌm/	drum	7. /mʌk/	muck
3. /kʌp/	cup	8. /mʌt/	mutt
4. /bʌst/	bust	9. /sʌn/	sun
5. /hʌg/	hug	10. /hʌmp/	hump

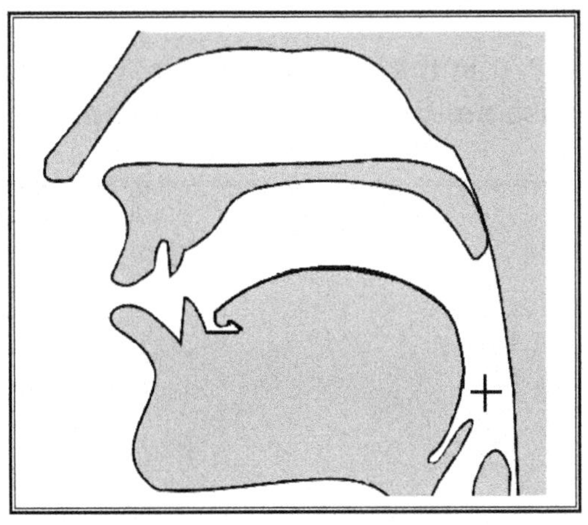

Fig. 4.14: (shwa)

/ə/ Keyword: *Above* /əˈbʌv/

Tongue height: Mid

Tongue position: Central

Degree of tongue tension: Lax

Degree of lip rounding: Unrounded

Common spellings beginning with the most commonly used (Hanna et al., 1966):

o:	Lemon
a:	Above
i:	Imitate
e:	Moment
u:	Circus
eo:	Luncheon
ie:	Conscience

Exercise 4.29 Transcribe the following words containing /ə/ in the first syllable, which is unstressed. Remember that all consonants in this exercise are the same as orthography:

1. away /əwe/
2. alone /əlon/
3. again /əgɛn/
4. across /əkrɔs/

Exercise 4.30 Transcribe the following words containing /ə/ in the second syllable, which is unstressed. Remember that all consonants in this exercise are the same as orthography:

1. sofa /sofə/
2. soda /sodə/
3. coma /komə/
4. gallop /gæləp/
5. okra /okrə/

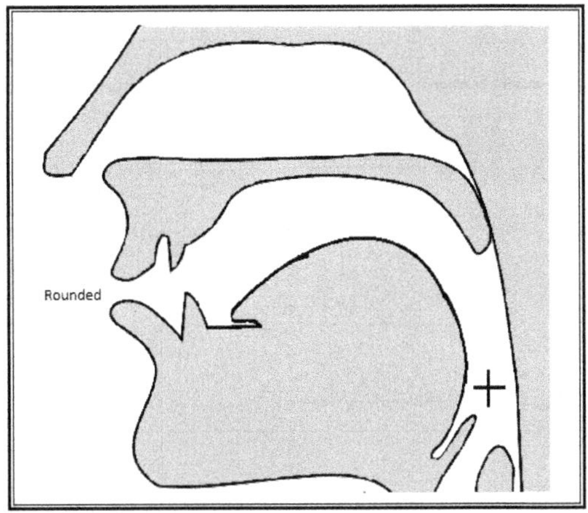

Fig. 4.15: 3r (bird)

/ɝ/ Keyword: *Bird* /bɝd/

Tongue height: Mid

Tongue position: Central

Degree of tongue tension: Tense

Degree of lip rounding: Rounded

Common spellings beginning with the most commonly used (Hanna et al., 1966):

er:	Fern
ur:	Murder
ir:	First
ear:	Earth
or:	Word
our:	Courage

Exercise 4.31 Transcribe the following words containing /ɝ/. Remember that all consonants in this exercise are the same as orthography:

1. burn	/bɝn/	6. girl	/gɝl/
2. first	/fɝst/	7. twirl	/twɝl/
3. irk	/ɝk/	8. fur	/fɝ/
4. sir	/sɝ/	9. purr	/pɝ/
5. dirt	/dɝt/	10. worm	/wɝm/

Exercise 4.32 Read the phonetic symbols to identify the following words:

1. /pɝk/	perk	6. /stɝ/	stir
2. /skɝt/	skirt	7. /kɝb/	curb
3. /wɝk/	work	8. /sɝv/	serve
4. /bɝst/	burst	9. /nɝd/	nerd
5. /lɝk/	lurk	10. /kɝs/	curse

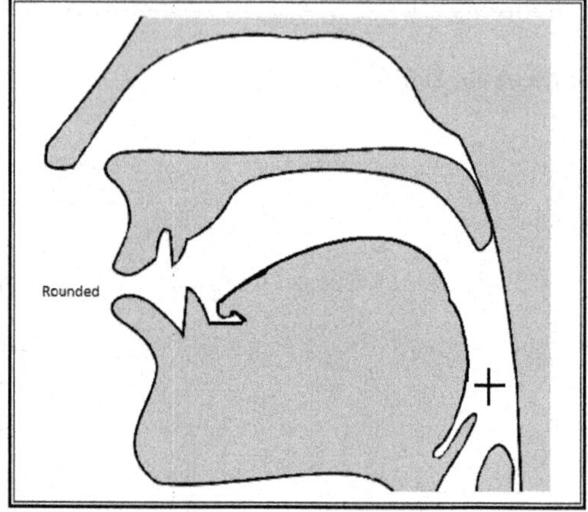

Fig. 4.16: er (father)

/ɚ/ Keyword: *Sister* /sɪstɚ/

Tongue height: Mid

Tongue position: Central

Degree of tongue tension: Lax

Degree of lip rounding: Rounded

Common spellings beginning with the most commonly used (Hanna et al., 1966):

er:	Father
or:	Liquor
ar:	Dollar
ir:	Confirmation
our:	Glamour
re:	Centre
ure:	Pleasure

Exercise 4.33 Transcribe the following words containing /ɚ/. Remember that all consonants in this exercise are the same as orthography:

1. sister /sɪstɚ/
2. butter /bətɚ/
3. bitter /bɪtɚ/
4. under /ʌndɚ/
5. over /ovɚ/

Exercise 4.34 Name each vowel:

1. Low, Front æ
2. Low-mid, Front ɛ
3. High, Back u
4. High-mid, Front ɪ
5. Mid-central, Tense, Rounded ɝ
6. Low-mid, Back ɔ
7. High, Front i
8. Unstressed Rhotic ɚ
9. Mid, Front e
10. Mid, Back o
11. Unstressed Neutral ə
12. Low, Back ɑ

Exercise 4.35 Transcribe all the vowels in the following words.

1. August	/ɔ, ə/
2. panda	/æ, ə/
3. delta	/ɛ, ə/
4. necessary	/ɛ, ə, ɛr, i/
5. attack	/ə, æ/
6. often	/ɔ, ɪ/
7. alert	/ə, ɝ/
8. cobra	/o, ə/
9. column	/ɑ, ə/
10. suffice	/ə, aɪ/

Exercise 4.36 Transcribe the front, central, and back vowels heard in the following words:

	Front		Central		Back	
1.	bead	/i/	bird	/ɝ/	bode	/o/
2.	pit	/ɪ/	putt	/ʌ/	put	/ʊ/
3.	pain	/e/	pun	/ʌ/	pawn	/ɔ/
4.	peg	/ɛ/	pug	/ʌ/	pog	/ɑ/
5.	cat	/æ/	curt	/ɝ/	caught	/ɔ/
6.	mat	/æ/	mutt	/ʌ/	moat	/o/
7.	ten	/ɛ/	turn	/ɝ/	tune	/u/
8.	gain	/e/	gun	/ʌ/	goon	/u/
9.	fin	/ɪ/	fun	/ʌ/	phone	/o/
10.	teen	/i/	tun	/ʌ/	tone	/o/

Diphthongs

When two successive vowel sounds are rapidly blended and function as a single phoneme, a diphthong is the result (Kent & Read, 2002). Like monothongs, diphthongs are produced with an unobstructed vocal tract. There are three types of diphthongs presented in this text:

Phonemic Diphthongs

Phonemic Diphthongs make a meaning contrast when produced. For example, the diphthongs in the words *coy* /kɔɪ/ and *cow* /kaʊ/ make a meaning distinction between the two words. Phonemic diphthongs cannot be reduced to a monophthong (Edwards, 2003). The four phonemic diphthongs introduced in this text are: /aɪ/, /aʊ/, /ɔɪ/, and /ju/.

Non-Phonemic Diphthongs

Non-Phonemic Diphthongs can be reduced to a monophthong. They are defined by stress and don't produce a meaning contrast (Edwards, 2003). There are two non-phonemic diphthongs: /eɪ/ as in the word *pay* and /oʊ/ as in the word *go*. These two diphthongs appear in strongly stressed syllables or may be used in certain dialects; however, they are not phonemically different from the monophthong versions; i.e., they don't result in a change in word meaning. For example, the word *bake* could be produced with either the monophthong /bek/ or the diphthong /beɪk/ and be recognized as the same word. This text will use the monophthong versions of these vowels exclusively; for example, *pay* will be transcribed /pe/ and *go* will be transcribed /go/.

Rhotic/Controlled /r/ Diphthongs and Triphthongs

Lax monophthongs combined with the r-controlled unstressed central vowel (schwar) result in rhotic or "r-colored" diphthongs. The lax monophthong will serve as the onglide, and the schwar will be the offglide (Edwards, 2003). There are five rhotic diphthongs presented in this text:

/ɑr/ as in *car* /kɑr/

/ɔr/ as in *core* /kɔr/

/ɪr/ as in *ear* /ɪr/

/ɛr/ as in *air* /ɛr/

/ʊr/ as in *tour* /tʊr/

In addition to the five rhotic diphthongs, there are two r-controlled triphthongs, which are produced by the rapid blending of a diphthong and the schwar. They are:

/aɪr/ as in *fire* /faɪr/

/aʊr/ as in *our* /aʊr/

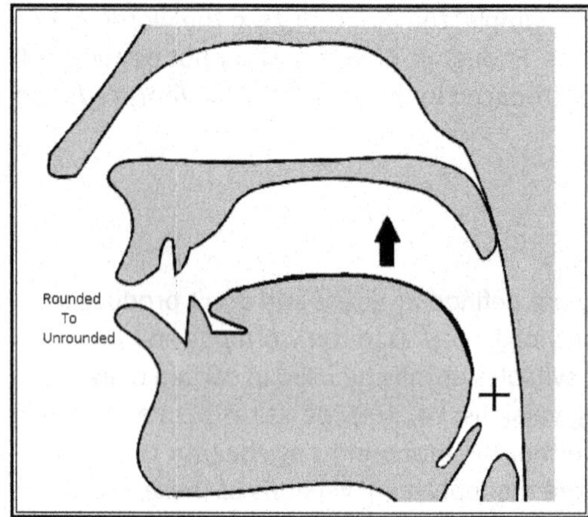

Fig. 4.17: oy

/ɔɪ/ Keyword: *Boy* /bɔɪ/

Rising Mid-Back to High Front Diphthong: Jaw begins in the mid-back rounded position (on-glide), and then rapidly moves to a high front unrounded position (off-glide) to form the single sound /ɔɪ/.

Common spellings beginning with the most commonly used (Hanna et al., 1966):

oi:	Foil
oy:	Toy
oi-e:	Noise

Exercise 4.37 Transcribe the following words containing /ɔɪ/. Remember that all consonants in this exercise are the same as orthography:

1. boy /bɔɪ/
2. soy /sɔɪ/
3. toy /tɔɪ/
4. voice /vɔɪs/
5. spoil /spɔɪl/

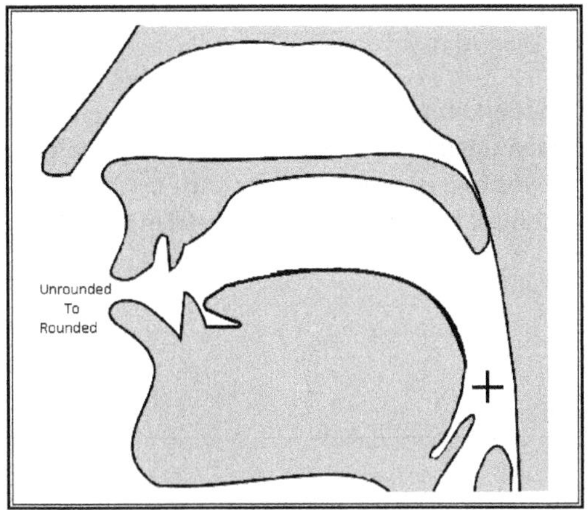

Fig. 4.18: ow

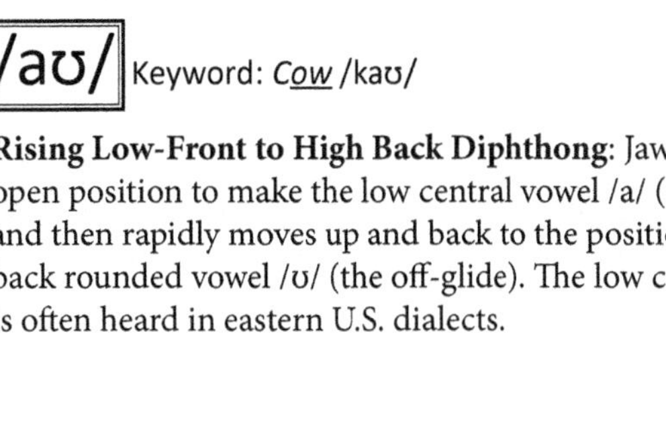

/aʊ/ Keyword: C<u>ow</u> /kaʊ/

Rising Low-Front to High Back Diphthong: Jaw begins in an open position to make the low central vowel /a/ (the on-glide) and then rapidly moves up and back to the position for the mid-back rounded vowel /ʊ/ (the off-glide). The low central vowel /a/ is often heard in eastern U.S. dialects.

Common spellings beginning with the most commonly used (Hanna et al., 1966):

ou:	Hound
ow:	How
hou:	Hour
ough:	Bough
ou-e:	Pounce

Exercise 4.38 Transcribe the following words containing /aʊ/. Remember that all consonants in this exercise are the same as orthography:

1. cow /kaʊ/
2. foul /faʊl/
3. now /naʊ/
4. doubt /daʊt/
5. wow /waʊ/

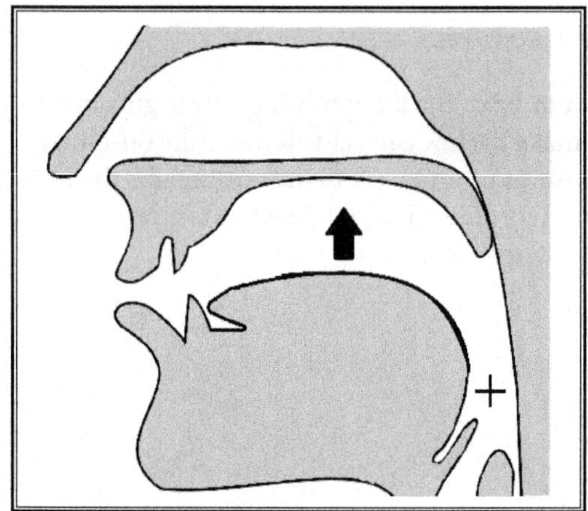
Fig. 4.19: ai

/aɪ/ Keyword: *Dive* /daɪv/

Rising Low-Front to High Front Diphthong: Jaw begins in an open position to make the low central vowel /a/ (the on-glide) and then rapidly moves to a high position for the /ɪ/ (the off-glide). The low central vowel /a/ is often heard in eastern U.S. dialects.

Common spellings beginning with the most commonly used (Hanna et al., 1966):

i:	Idea
i-e:	Time
ye:	Eye
eigh:	Height
igh:	Thigh
ui:	Guide

Exercise 4.39 Transcribe the following words containing /aɪ/. Remember that all consonants in this exercise are the same as orthography:

1. knife /naɪf/
2. tight /taɪt/
3. might /maɪt/
4. life /laɪf/
5. strife /straɪf/

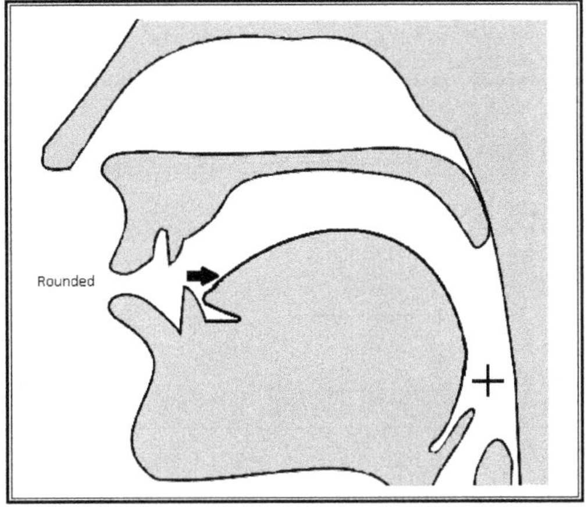

Fig. 4.20: ju

/ju/ Keyword: You /ju/

High-Front to High-Back Diphthong: Jaw begins in a somewhat open position to make the /j/ and then rapidly moves up and back to the position for the high rounded vowel /u/.

Common spellings beginning with the most commonly used (Hanna et al., 1966):

u:	Unit
u-e:	Cute
eau:	Beauty
ew:	Pew
hu:	Humor
ut:	Debut
you:	You

Exercise 4.40 Transcribe the following words containing /ju/. Remember that all consonants in this exercise are the same as orthography:

1. muse /mjuz/
2. fuze /fjuz/
3. fume /fjum/
4. used /juzd/
5. few /fju/

Exercise 4.41 Transcribe the diphthongs in the following words:

1. how	/aʊ/	14. pie	/aɪ/
2. mine	/aɪ/	15. prowl	/aʊ/
3. joy	/ɔɪ/	16. I	/aɪ/
4. high	/aɪ/	17. ointment	/ɔɪ/
5. now	/aʊ/	18. choice	/ɔɪ/
6. Roy	/ɔɪ/	19. plough	/aʊ/
7. bite	/aɪ/	20. oil	/ɔɪ/
8. crown	/aʊ/	21. oyster	/ɔɪ/
9. use	/ju/	22. eyes	/aɪ/
10. toy	/ɔɪ/	23. you	/ju/
11. dice	/aɪ/	24. ice	/aɪ/
12. cloud	/aʊ/	25. owl	/aʊ/
13. hound	/aʊ/	26. mouse	/aʊ/
27. ouch	/aʊ/	34. cute	/ju/
28. time	/aɪ/	35. poise	/ɔɪ/
29. sigh	/aɪ/	36. ounce	/aʊ/
30. outside	/aʊ/, /aɪ/	37. boy	/ɔɪ/
31. house	/aʊ/	38. avoid	/ɔɪ/
32. lie	/aɪ/	39. hide	/aɪ/
33. about	/aʊ/	40. beauty	/ju/

Rhotic Diphthongs

For these diphthongs, the /r/ phoneme that follows a lax monophthong "colors" and changes the vowel's quality, thus creating what are termed "rhotic" or "r-colored" diphthongs. The lax monophthong serves as the on-glide, and the central vowel (schwar) serves as the off-glide. Some refer to these as "centering diphthongs" as opposed to rhotic diphthongs (Van Riper & Smith, 1979).

/ɑr/ Keyword: C<u>ar</u> /ɑr/

/ɔr/ Keyword: D<u>oor</u> /dɔr/

/ɛr/ Keyword: P<u>ear</u> /pɛr/

/ɪr / Keyword: <u>Ear</u> /ɪr/

/ʊr/ Keyword: P<u>oor</u> /pʊr/

Rhotic Triphthongs

Rhotic triphthongs are created when a diphthong is produced in rapid succession, creating one sound. The two triphthongs are:

/aɪr/: Keyword: *<u>fire</u>* /faɪr/

/aʊr/: Keyword: *<u>our</u>*/aʊr/

Note: Sometimes the r-controlled diphthongs and triphthongs are transcribed with the schwar /ɚ/ instead of the /r/. Regardless which symbol is used, the sound functions as a vowel in words. For example:

/ɑr/→ /ɑɚ/	/ʊr/→/ʊɚ/
/ɔr/ → /ɔɚ/	/aɪr/→/aɪɚ/
/ɪr/ →/ɪɚ/	/aʊr/→/aʊɚ

Exercise 4.42 Transcribe the rhotic diphthongs and triphthongs in the following words:

1. square	/ɛr/	16. choir	/aɪr/
2. dire	/aɪr/	17. pork	/ɔr/

3. board	/ɔr/	18. mare	/ɛr/
4. hair	/ɛr/	19. beer	/ɪr/
5. bear	/ɛr/	20. cork	/ɔr/
6. tore	/ɔr/	21. tour	/ʊr/
7. hour	/aʊr/	22. ear	/ɪr/
8. tire	/aɪr/	23. card	/ar/
9. pier	/ɪr/	24. beard	/ɪr/
10. arm	/ar/	25. fear	/ɪr/
11. deer	/ɪr/	26. barn	/ar/
12. four	/ɔr/	27. our	/aʊr/
13. store	/ɔr/	28. heir	/ɛr/
14. stare	/ɛr/	29. clear	/ɪr/
15. pear	/ɛr/	30. tier	/ɪr/
31. dare	/ɛr/	36. park	/ar/
32. mar	/ar/	37. pier	/ɪr/
33. star	/ar/	38. dare	/ɛr/
34. mire	/aɪr/	39. fair	/ɛr/
35. poise	/ɔɪ/	40. glare	/ɛr/

CONCLUSION

Most vowels can be described in terms of the frequencies of their first two formants. Formants are resonances in the vocal tract that result from the specific gestures of our articulators. The first formant is influenced by the position of the tongue within the oral cavity, and the second formant is affected by the height of the tongue. The importance of vowels cannot be overestimated—vowels are the nucleus of our syllables and the power of our speech—vowels are what make speech possible.

CHAPTER

Previous chapters have introduced the importance of consonants and vowels and how these segmental units form spoken words. Chapter 4 highlighted vowels and their function as the nucleus of syllables. This chapter's focus is the suprasegmentals or prosodic features: stress and intonation. These prosodic properties are expressed in spoken language as an "overlay" to the speech sounds being articulated (Gerken & McGregor, 1998). Stress was introduced in the third chapter's discussion of its effect on central vowels. This chapter will be concerned with both stress and intonation in relation to connected speech and how these components impact communication.

SUPRASEGMENTALS

Phonemes are considered segmental units; however, speech is not just guided by phonemes. When segmental units form words and words, in turn, form connected speech, much meaning is conveyed through the use of suprasegmentals (Gerken & McGregor, 1998), which serve to form an overlay of prosodic properties attached to sound segments. Stress and intonation are the suprasegmental features that will be discussed in this chapter, and they work together to contribute meaning to our spoken messages. These properties are used simultaneously with phonetic segments and can indicate a variety of information vital to communication.

Lexical Stress

As discussed in Chapter 3, stress denotes syllable prominence, and it is primarily the vowel segment that is stressed, because vowels form the nucleus of syllables. There are many factors that interact that differentiate a stressed syllable from an unstressed one:

1. Loudness: A stressed syllable will be louder than an unstressed one.
2. Length: A stressed syllable will be longer in duration than an unstressed one.
3. Pitch: A stressed syllable will be produced with higher pitch than an unstressed one.

Stress can be thought of as the interplay of pitch, loudness, and length. Fry (1955) proposed that of the above features, higher pitch was the most influential perceptual cue in English when signaling syllable prominence. Ladefoged (2005) noted the role of vocal fold tension and the amount of air passing through the folds to produce stressed syllables. The act of expelling air from the lungs causes larger and, thus, louder amplitude of vocal fold vibration, which, in turn, increases the pitch, thereby making the syllable longer and more prominent.

Because stress is a particularly complex feature and because it is relative, there are four degrees of stress that are linguistically applicable in English:

Primary

The most prominent syllable. Every word regardless of how many syllables will have one and only one syllable with primary stress. In the International Phonetic Alphabet (IPA), the upper mark /ˈ/ is used to indicate primary stress.

Secondary

The second most prominent syllable. This syllable receives more stress relative to unstressed syllables in the word, but not as much stress as the primary stressed syllable. In English, depending on word length, there may be more than one incidence of secondary stress. Secondary stress will always precede primary stress. The lower mark /ˌ/ is used to indicate secondary stress.

Tertiary

The third most prominent syllable. This syllable will contain a full vowel, i.e. the vowel will not be reduced to the schwa. There is no marking in IPA to indicate tertiary stress.

None

Weak syllable that contains a reduced vowel, i.e. the schwa. There is no marking in IPA to indicate a weak syllable containing no stress.

To demonstrate the above levels of stress, we will use a word you no doubt have become very familiar with from reading this chapter: *Suprasegmental*. Suprasegmental has five syllables which demonstrate the four levels of stress. Consider the following levels:

Primary: Su-pra-seg-**men**-tal

Secondary: **Su**-pra-seg-men-tal

Tertiary: Su-pra-**seg**-men-tal

None: Su-**pra**-seg-men-**tal**

The IPA transcription of *suprasegmental* showing its stress is as follows: /ˌsuprəsɛgˈmɛntl̩/. Note that the syllable receiving primary stress is marked, as is the syllable receiving secondary stress. The syllable receiving tertiary stress is /sɛg/. It is less stressed than the other two, but still contains the full vowel /ɛ/. Also note, that the two syllables without stress contain a schwa vowel /prə/ or a syllabic consonant /l̩/ (Syllabic consonants are always unstressed). One final word—no English word will start with two consecutive syllables that contain either tertiary or no stress; the *supragegmental* example above illustrates this, as well.

Determining stress can be a difficult task for students just learning word stress. The following is an adaptation of rules related to stress from Pennington Publishing Blog, June 2010, English Language Rules Governing Primary Stress.

Stress Rule #1: Two or more syllable words will have a syllable containing a stressed or primary vowel that indicates that syllable is to be read with greater emphasis or stress than the remaining syllable(s). Example, *for-gíve.*

Stress Rule #2: All words have only one syllable containing a vowel with primary stress. *Some* words may have one or more syllables requiring secondary or less emphasized stress. This is true especially for long words. Example, *iˌn-vi-ta'-tion.*

Stress Rule #3: A word that contains a root before a double consonant usually has a primary stress that falls on the vowel before the double consonant. Example, *rún-ning*

Stress Rule #4: A word containing a monothong will sometimes be reduced to the schwa /ə/. This syllable will always be unstressed. Example, *a-bóve.*

Stress Rule #5: Primary stress usually falls on the first syllable of a two-syllable word. Example, èv-en.

Stress Rule #6: In a two syllable word that has a prefix followed by a root, the stress usually falls on the root. Example, *dis-gúst.*

Stress Rule #7: A two syllable word that functions as either a noun or a verb usually has the primary stress fall on the first syllable of nouns and the second syllable of verbs. Examples, *re'c-ord as a noun ; re-co'rd as a verb.*

Stress Rule #8: A three-syllable word for which the first syllable is a root usually has primary stress on the first syllable. Example, *strúc-tur-al.*

Stress Rule #9: Three-syllable words made up of prefix-root-suffix usually have a primary stress on the second syllable. Example, *con-tént-ment.*

Stress Rule #10: Four-syllable words usually have primary stress on the second syllable. Example, *re-vér-si-ble.*

Another "trick" in determining the stressed syllable of a multisyllabic word is to insert an expletive into the word. We intuitively will insert the expletive before the stressed syllable. Below are some examples of this "trick," and because this is a "family-friendly" text, I will use *freaking* as my expletive. Notice how natural it is to insert the expletive before the stressed syllable.

- ab-so –*freaking*-LUTE-ly
- fan-*freaking*- TAS-tic
- gua-ran-*freaking*-TEE
- hy-per-*freaking*-TEN-sion

Lexical stress is the stress placed on a syllable in a word. Every word will have a stressed syllable with the vowel receiving the stress. In English, stress is also sometimes used to discern between nouns and verbs. Lexical stress is part of a word's pronunciation and can be used to differentiate similar words. Do you want a ***record*** of the event, or do you want to ***record*** a person's statement? The syllable stress on these words along with contextual cues aid meaning.

Students often find determining word stress a difficult task. The following is a list of bolded bisyllabic words that are used as either a noun or a verb dependent on the sentence context, and each will have different syllable stress contingent on how it is being used. Read each example aloud to determine the proper word stress. This exercise should aid in helping with syllable stress identification.

Underline the stressed syllable in each bolded word.

Verb	Noun
Drinking will **impact** your ability to drive.	The **impact** of drinking affects driving.
She must **increase** her bid.	The **increase** in my pay was significant.
Did you **insert** the photo in the book?	Here is the magazine **insert**.
Please **permit** her to miss class.	My parking **permit** was too expensive.
We must **produce** more oil.	We bought **produce** at the market.
You **protest** too much.	There is a **protest** on Dickson Street.
Transport the livestock to the sale barn.	I need **transport** to the airport.
I won't **subject** you to my singing.	My favorite **subject** is phonology.
Don't **insult** my intelligence.	Her **insult** hurt my feelings.
Our hard work will **impact** the results.	What is the **impact** of our contribution.
Please **increase** my salary.	The **increase** in my salary will help.
I hope this doesn't **conflict** with the time.	There's a **conflict** with your appointment.

I will **contest** the results.	The **contest** lasts until next week.
I will **invite** him.	Thanks for the **invite** to your party!
Contrast the two points of view.	The new paint color adds a nice **contrast**.
I will **display** the awards.	The awards make a nice **display**.

As has been previously mentioned, determining the primary stress of syllables can be, uh, stressful for students. The following are examples of several multisyllabic words in which different syllables are stressed. Read these examples, complete the exercise, and try not to get too stressed.

Words with stress on the first syllable

AL	*cohol*		/ˈælkəˌhɔl/
AT	*mos*	*phere*	/ˈætmosˌfɪr/
CAL	*ci*	*um*	/ˈkælˌsiəm/
CA	*ta*	*lyst*	/ˈkædəˌlɪst/
DI	*a*	*gram*	/ˈdaɪəˌgræm/
DOC	*tor*		/ˈdacˌtɚ/
HAN	*di*	*cap*	/ˈhændiˌkæp/

TES	*ti*	*mo*	*ny*
CAP	*i*	*tal*	*ism*

Bisyllabic words with stress on the second syllable

a	*BOUT*
in	*CLUDE*
ma	*CHINE*
a	*WAY*
him	*SELF*
su	*PPORT*
re	*VIEW*
a	*GREE*
with	*IN*
be	*CAUSE*

Trisyllabic words with stress on the second syllable

spe	CIF	ic /ˌspəˈsɪfɪc/
eco	NOM	ic /ˌɛkoˈnamɪk/
con	DI	tion /ˌkənˈdɪʃɪn/
defi	NI	tion /ˌdɛfɪˈnɪʃɪn/
com	PU	ter /ˌcəmˈputɚ/
i	CON	ic /ˌaɪˈkanɪk/
nu	TRI	tion /ˌnuˈtrɪʃɪn/
ad	VI	sor /ˌæedˈvaɪsɚ/
co	VA	lent /ˌkəˈvelɪnt/
ro	TA	tion /ˌroˈteʃɪn/

Words with stress next to the last syllable

con	*fron*	***TA***	*tion*
hy	*per*	***TEN***	*sion*
ex	*pec*	***TA***	*tion*
ma	*ture*	***RA***	*tion*
hy	*ber*	***NA***	*tion*
ac	*ti*	***VA***	*tion*

Based on what you have learned about stress, underline the syllable that receives primary stress in the following words:

expert	demand	July
attempt	information	water
amount	composer	expensive
rescue	country	reply
defense	argue	gorilla

remainder	system	central
mental	effect	remember
detective	research	increase
demand	December	machine
control	number	problem
departure	complain	engine
disease	emotion	another
eclipse	barracuda	accommodation
canal	expect	presentation

Prosodic Stress

As has been discussed, **lexical stress** has to do with stress placed on syllables, while **prosodic stress**, on the other hand, relates to stress on a sentence as a whole. In phrases and sentences, some words are stressed more than others. Instead of changing the individual meaning of words, prosodic stress will alter the connotation of sentences or phrases (Ladefoged, 2005). Placing stress on different words in a sentence will convey different meanings. For example, in the sentence, *"I didn't go to Arkansas,"* consider the following:

Example 1: *"**I** didn't go to Arkansas."* In this sentence, the speaker is stating that *she* was not the one who went to Arkansas.

Example 2: *"I **didn't** go to Arkansas."* In this sentence, the speaker is stating that perhaps she was planning on going but *didn't* go to Arkansas.

Example 3: *"I didn't go to **Arkansas**."* In this sentence, the speaker is stating that *Arkansas* was not the place where she went.

Intonation

As has been discussed, pitch is a component of word stress and roughly corresponds to the acoustic feature of fundamental frequency, i.e., the vibration of the vocal folds. Pitch allows for the placing of sounds on a scale ranging from low to high. In connected speech, different segments in an utterance will be produced in different pitches, i.e., there will be patterns of rises and falls; this pitch variation is known as intonation (O'Grady, Archibald, Aronoff, Rees-Miller, 2001). Sentence meaning is often dependent on intonation patterns, such as indicating whether one is making a statement or asking a question. Note these examples:

Rising

A rise in intonation can denote a variety of different meanings. It can indicate that one is questioning, surprised, doubtful, or hesitant, to name just a few. In other words, intonation patterns contribute much meaning to our spoken messages.

Falling

Falling intonation patterns also signal meaning. Used in making declarative sentences (statements), these patterns are the most common type in English. Falling intonation patterns are also used when making imperative sentences (commands), or when producing exclamatory sentences.

Note the following examples:

1. *"I hurt your feelings."* If these words are stated with a falling pitch, the speaker is simply making a statement; he is admitting that he hurt his communication partner's feelings.
2. *"I hurt your feelings?"* These words spoken with a rise in pitch toward the end of the utterance, will signal that the speaker is asking for clarification whether or not the communication partner's feelings were hurt.
3. *"**I** hurt your feelings?"* If these words are produced with both a rise in intonation at the end of the utterance and prosodic stress on the word *"I,"* then the speaker is questioning whether *he* was the one who hurt the communication partner's feelings.

CONCLUSION

It is easy to see from this chapter's discussion of stress and intonation the important role that suprasegmental properties play in aiding communication. Without these vital features, speech would not only be difficult to understand, but it would also be unfocused, monotone, and uninteresting—additionally the bulk of speaker intent would be lost.

CHAPTER

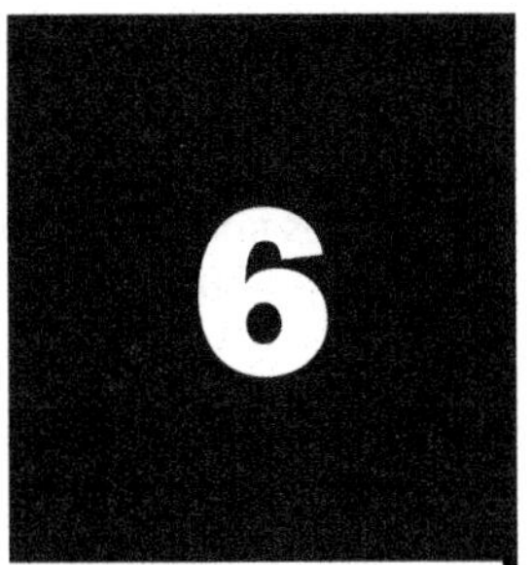

Chapter 4 discussed the importance that vowels play in human communication. Vowels provide the power to our utterances, and without them, speech would not be possible. Consonants, too, play a vital role, because they provide intelligibility to our speech. Recall that there are similarities in vowel production—there are vowels produced with the tongue in different portions of the mouth and with the tongue at varying heights—there are also similarities and differences in the ways in which consonants are produced. Being able to recognize the characteristics of phonemes is a vital skill for the speech-language pathologist (SLP) in analyzing speech, diagnosing disorders, and developing treatment plans. This chapter introduces the different ways in which phonemes are classified. You will be introduced to the many aspects that phonemes have in common and the features that differentiate them. Later, in Chapter 10, which deals with transcribing the speech of children with phonological disorders, you will put this knowledge to use by analyzing disordered speech.

CLASSIFICATION SCHEMES

Consonants differ from vowels in terms of the comparative openness of the vocal tract and how they function within syllables. Recall in Chapter 4 that vowels are produced with an open vocal tract; consonants, however, are described by the degree of constriction or closure of the vocal tract and the location within the vocal tract where the constriction or closure occurs. Additionally, all vowels are produced with vocal fold vibration, whereas not all consonants are produced with voicing. Although vowels are identified by the first two or three formant frequencies, consonants are typically described in terms of the manner in which they are produced, the place within the vocal tract where they are produced, and whether or not they are made with vocal fold vibration (Van Riper & Smith, 1979).

There are two major classification schemes that are beneficial to SLPs when treating communication disorders: the **Classical Classification System** and the **Distinctive Features**. These schemes not only help in the understanding of phonemes, they also afford information that is vital in diagnosis and treatment, because they provide the basis for many assessments and therapeutic interventions.

Classical Classification System

The **Classical Classification System** uses three parameters to classify consonants: **Manner**, **Place**, and **Voice**. **Manner** will be discussed first and refers to "how" the speech sound is produced. More specifically, manner indicates the way in which the airstream is modified to produce phonemes and the degree of constriction or closure during production (Van Riper & Smith, 1979). In terms of **manner**, there are two major categories of how speech sounds are produced, **obstruents** and **sonorants**.

Manner

Obstruents

As the name implies, there is some degree of "obstruction" or constriction within the vocal tract that impedes the airstream for the three different types of obstruents. The **obstruents** (Ohde & Sharf, 1992) include **stops, fricatives,** and **affricates.**

Stops

The manner of sounds produced with the airflow completely stopped within the vocal tract and then released. Shriberg and Kent (1995) described an audible burst of noise heard upon release of the stop closure. They further portrayed the closing and opening movements for the stops to be the fastest movements in speech. There are two phases for production of the stops: Phase 1 — the air is stopped somewhere in the oral cavity, and Phase 2—the air is suddenly released. The velopharyngeal port is closed during production. Sometimes the phonemes for this manner of articulation are referred to as "plosives" or "stop-plosives"; in this text, they will be referred to as "stops." There are six stops: /p b t d k g/. The phonemes /p b/, /t d/, /k g/ are cognate pairs, meaning they share the same manner and place of articulation but differ in voicing. The stops are as follows:

/p/ as in "pit" /pɪt/
/b/ as in "bit" /bɪt/
/t/ as in "tip" /tɪp/
/d/ as in "dip" /dɪp/
/k/ as in "came" /kem/
/g/ as in "game" /gem/

Fricatives

The manner of sounds that are produced by the airflow being forced through a narrow constriction somewhere in the vocal tract causing an audible turbulence that is characteristic of fricatives. Like the stops, the velopharyngeal port is closed during production. There are nine fricatives /s z f v ʃ ʒ θ ð h/ and four pairs of fricative cognates /s z/, /f v/, / ʃ ʒ/, and /θ ð/. The /h/ is the only fricative that is not part of a cognate. The fricatives are:

/s/ as in "sip" /sɪp/
/z/ as in "zip" /zɪp/
/f/ as in "fat" /fæt/
/v/ as in "vat" /væt/
/ʃ/ as in "Ship" /ʃɪp/
/ʒ/ as in "beige" /beʒ/
/θ/ as in "think" /θɪŋk/
/ð/ as in "this" /ðɪs/
/h/ as in "hat" /hæt/

Affricates

The manner of sounds that are a blend of a stop phoneme and a fricative phoneme. The term "affricate" means "a blend." There are two affricates, the cognates /ʧ/ and /ʤ/. For the production of the affricates the stop component occurs first with complete closure between two articulators, but instead of a quick release like the plosive phase of a stop, the affricates are released gradually and with frication like a fricative. Like the stops and the fricatives, the velopharyngeal port is closed during production of the affricates. The affricates are:

/ʧ/ as in "Chip" /ʧɪp/
/ʤ/ as in "Judge" /ʤʌʤ/

Additionally, both affricates and the fricatives that are produced with high frequency turbulence can be grouped in a sound class known as **stridents**. The **stridents** include eight sounds: /f/, /v/, /s/, /z/, /ʃ/, /ʒ/, /ʧ/ and /ʤ/ but do not include the fricatives /h/, /θ/, and /ð/. The **sibilants** are high frequency sounds that have a more strident quality and longer duration than other consonants (Ohde & Sharf, 1992) and include six sounds: /s/, /z/, /ʃ/, /ʒ/, /ʧ/ and /ʤ/. The sibilants do not include the stridents /f/ and /v/.

Sonorants

Sonorant consonants are made with a relatively unobstructed vocal tract, are characterized by alterations of resonating cavities, and are of a vowel-like quality. Like vowels, sonorant consonants are always voiced and are defined by their formant frequencies (Ohde & Sharf, 1992). There are three different types of sonorant consonants: **liquids, glides,** and **nasals**. The **liquids** and the **glides** are considered "oral resonants" and are produced with the velopharyngeal port closed; conversely, the **nasals** are "nasal resonants" and are produced with the velopharyngeal port open, allowing coupling of the oral and nasal cavities.

Liquids

There are two types of liquids, the **lateral /l/** and the **rhotic /r/**. The two liquids, along with the glides (which will be discussed next), are considered "approximants," meaning that the primary articulators involved in their production only approximate without producing friction or blockage of the airflow. This manner of articulation produces a vowel-like quality. Both the liquid and the glide approximants will be produced with the velopharyngeal port closed. Unlike the glides, a fixed articulatory position is taken for the liquids. The lateral (meaning side) /l/ liquid is produced with the tongue blocking the center of the mouth while the airflow passes over the "sides" of the tongue. The tip of the tongue touches the alveolar ridge. The second type of liquid, /r/, is an approximate that is considered rhotic, which means it has an "r" timbre. There is much individual variation in production of the /r/ phoneme and many allophonic variations resulting from coarticulation. These aspects will be discussed later in this text. Like the /l/, the /r/ is an oral resonant typically produced with the tongue root retracted into the pharynx and the tongue body raised and retracted or tightly "bunched." However, there is great individual variation in the articulation of this complex sound. The International Phonetic Alphabet (IPA) symbols representing the liquids are identical to those of orthography.

/l/ as in "lip" /lɪp/
/r/ as in "rip" /rɪp/

Glides

Glides are very similar to liquids in that they are characterized by changes of resonating cavities, rather than constriction or blockage of the oral airstream. The glides are considered the most vowel-like phonemes of the approximants. Instead of a fixed articulatory position like that of the liquids, glides are defined by a rapid shift in placement, transitioning from a somewhat closed to a more open position. The vowel that follows the glide will determine how open the position of the glide will be. There are two glides (also called semi-vowels):

/j/ as in "yet" /jɛt/
/w/ as in "wet" /wɛt/

Nasals

The nasal consonants are produced in a manner very similar to that of the stop consonants, in that the airstream is completely obstructed within the oral cavity. The nasal /m/ has the same place of obstruction as the /p/ and /b/ stops, which are bilabial. The nasal /n/ airflow is impeded at the alveolar ridge like the /t/ and /d/ stops. Lastly, the production of the/ŋ/ is characterized by obstruction of the airflow at the velum, similar to that of the /k/ and /g/ stops. Unlike the stop phonemes, however, the nasal sounds are produced by lowering the velum, which allows for a coupling of the cavities. Instead of the air pressure being released through the oral cavities, like the stops, the voiced airstream and acoustic vibrations continually flow through the nasal cavity and out the nose. Unlike other manners of phoneme production, nasals are described by the velopharyngeal port opening, rather than the closing. The three nasal consonants are:

/m/ as in "mop" /mɑp/
/n/ as in "nip" /nɪp/
/ŋ/ as in "sing"

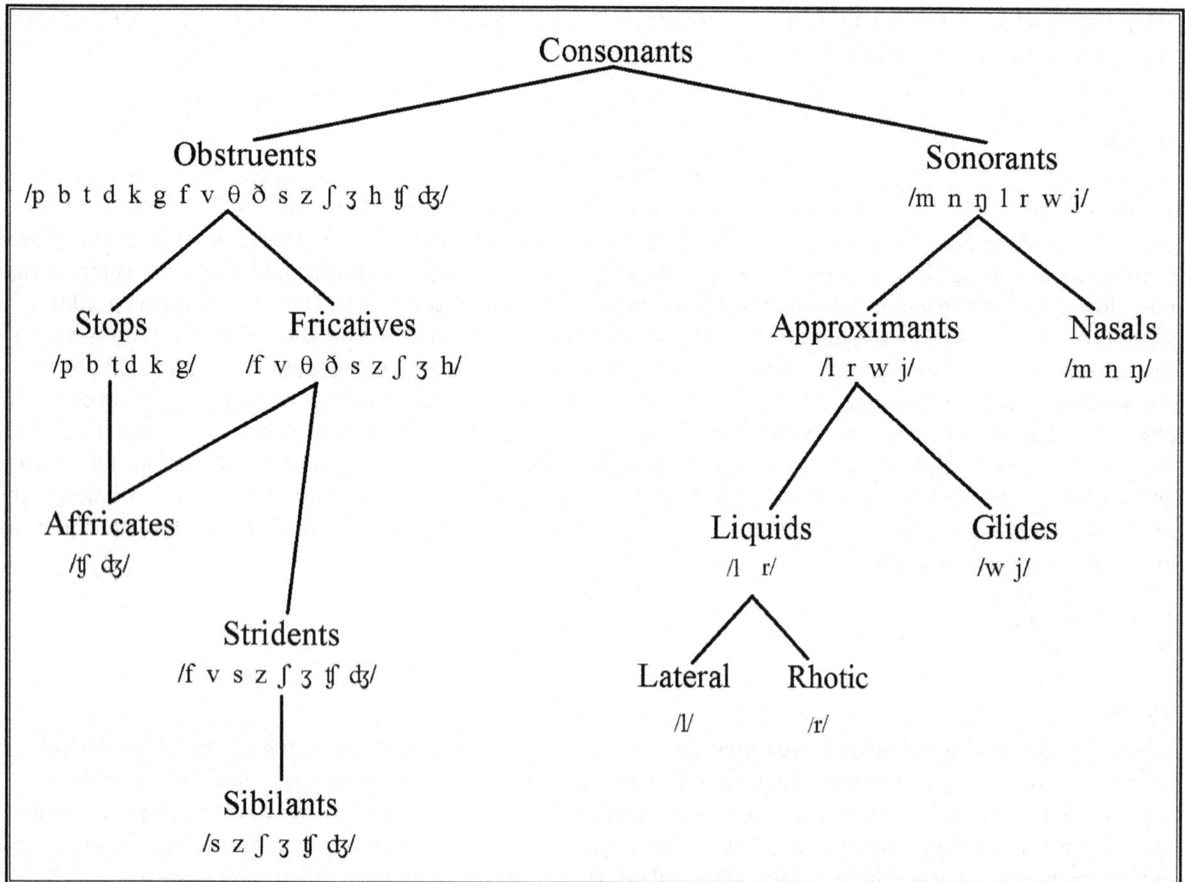

Fig. 6.1a: Consonant Tree

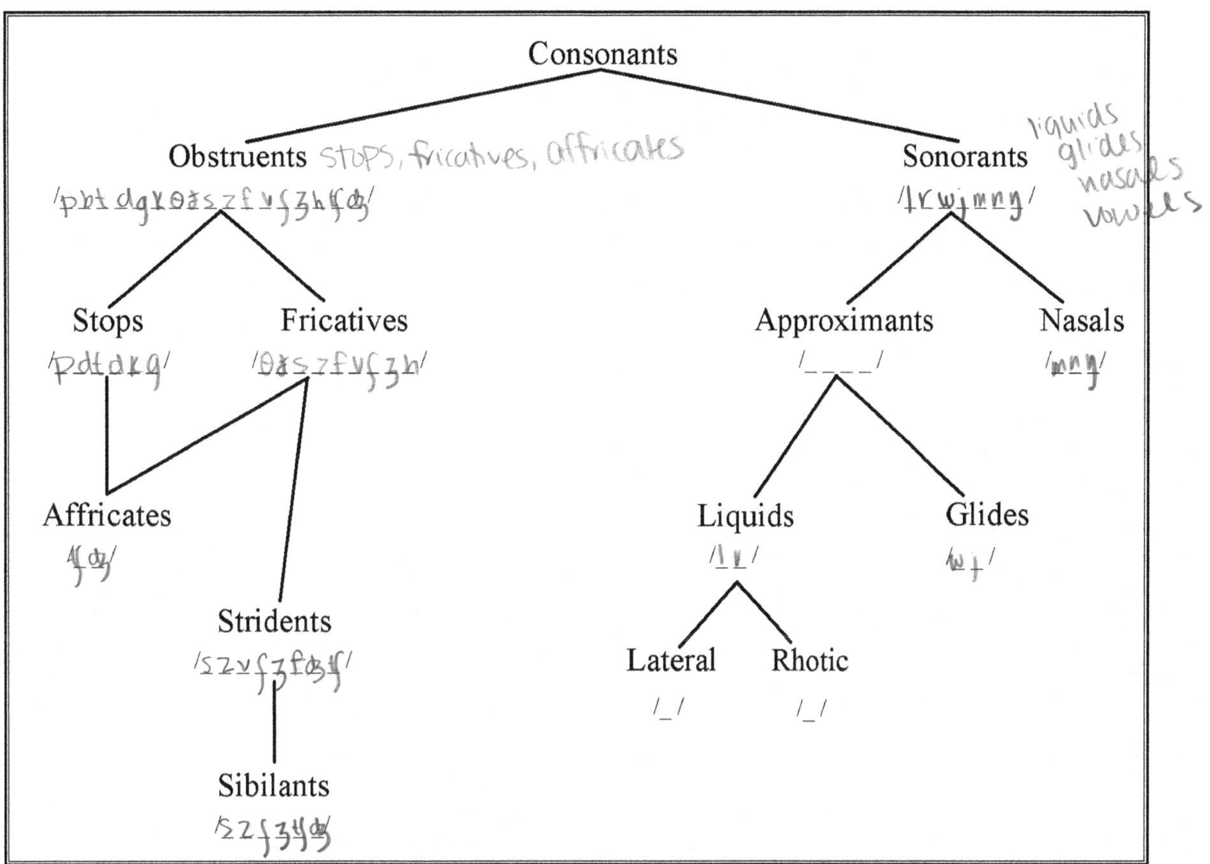

Fig. 6.1b: Blank Consonant Tree

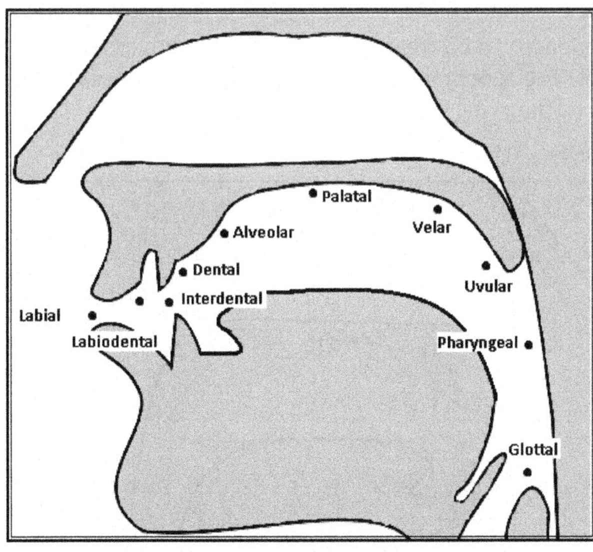

Fig. 6.2: Mouth Placement Diagram

Place

Next, we will discuss the second parameter of the classical classification system, **place** of articulation. From the lips to the glottis, **place** of articulation describes the point along the vocal tract where the focus of airflow blockage or constriction occurs in the production of speech sounds. **Place** describes "where" the phoneme is shaped. The following is a description of the places of articulation and the corresponding phonemes.

Bilabial

Bilabial, meaning "two lips," describes the most anterior place of articulation. Sounds made at this location will engage both of the lips. Bilabial sounds include: /p/, /b/, /m/ and /w/.

Labio-Dental

This placement describes sounds made with the bottom edge of the upper central incisors making contact with the bottom lips. The labio-dental sounds include /f/ and /v/.

Lingua-Dental (Interdental)

This placement indicates sounds made with the tongue touching the bottom edge of the upper incisors. The two lingua-dental sounds are /θ/ and /ð/.

Lingua-Alveolar

Refers to the tongue making partial or complete contact with the place immediately behind the upper central incisors known as the alveolar ridge. The lingua-alveolar sounds include /t/, /d/, /n/, /s/, /z/, and /l/.

Lingua-Palatal

This placement refers to the tongue contacting some portion of the hard palate (roof of the mouth). The hard palate lies just posterior to the alveolar ridge. Sounds considered palatal include /ʃ/, /ʒ/, /j/, /r/, and the alveo-palatals/ʧ/and/ʤ/. The /ʧ/ and /ʤ/ start at the alveolar ridge and end at the hard palate but are also considered "palatal" sounds.

Lingua-Velar

This place of articulation describes the tongue coming into contact with the velum, which is posterior to the hard palate and is located at the back of the oral cavity. The velar sounds include /k/ /g/ and /ŋ/.

Glottal

The glottis is the opening between the vocal folds, and turbulence can be created in this area when the folds are partially adducted. The fricative /h/ is produced at the glottis. The allophone glottal stop [ʔ] is also produced at the glottis, but it is produced by a complete stoppage of airflow by the vocal folds.

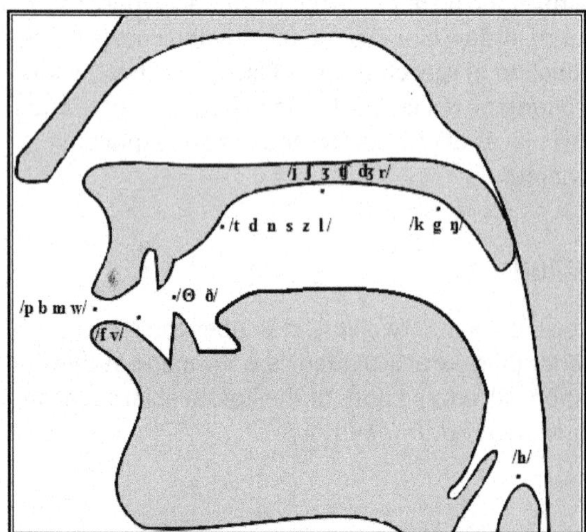

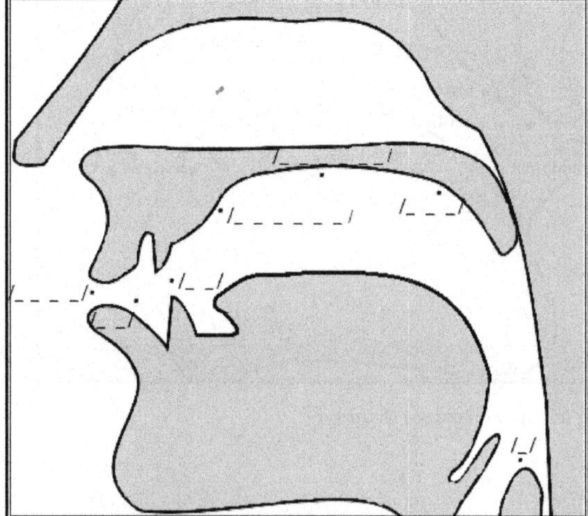

Fig. 6.3a-b: Placement Diagram

Voice

Voice is the third parameter by which consonants can be classified using the Classical Classification System. Consonants can be produced with voicing, i.e., vocal fold vibration, or they can be produced with no voicing, i.e., voiceless. All sonorants (including the vowels) are voiced, but the obstruents contain voiced and voiceless cognate pairs with the exception of the voiceless fricative /h/.

Manner:	Voicing:	Place:						
		Bilabial	Labiodental	Interdental	Alveolar	Palatal	Velar	Glottal
Stop	Voiceless	/p/			/t/		/k/	
	Voiced	/b/			/d/		/g/	
Fricative	Voiceless		/f/	/θ/	/s/	/ʃ/		/h/
	Voiced		/v/	/ð/	/z/	/ʒ/		
Affricate	Voiceless					/tʃ/		
	Voiced					/dʒ/		
Nasal	Voiced	/m/			/n/		/ŋ/	
(Liquid) Lateral	Voiced				/l/			
(Liquid) Rhotic	Voiced					/r/		
Glide	Voiced	/w/				/j/		

Fig. 6.4: Manner, Place, Voicing Chart

Distinctive Features

An alternate method of describing phonemes is by their **distinctive features**. Jakobson, Fant and Halle (1952) were the first to propose the idea that phonemes are a compilation of a set of indivisible acoustic and articulatory components termed distinctive features. There are many distinctive feature systems, but the method that is commonly used in speech-language pathology is the one proposed by the linguists Chomsky and Halle (1968). In this system, the features are presented in a binary fashion in which they are either (+) present or (-) absent for each phoneme. This system not only advances our grasp of the nature of phonemes, but it also aides in organizing sounds into sound classes. Like the Classical Classification System, the understanding of distinctive features is vital for SLPs, because the terms and concepts are rooted not only in our assessment instruments but also in our therapeutic interventions as well. The features listed below are an adaptation of the work of Chomsky and Halle (1968).

Obstruent

Sounds that are made with considerable constriction of the vocal tract that "obstructs" the airstream to some degree. The (+) obstruent sounds include the stops /p b t d k g/, the fricatives / s z f v ʃ ʒ Θ ð h/, and the affricates /ʧ ʤ/.

Sonorant

Sounds produced with a relatively open vocal tract so that the vocal folds vibrate spontaneously, and resonance is facilitated. The sonorant sounds include the liquids /l r/, glides /w j/, and nasals /m n ŋ/, and all vowels.

Consonantal

Sounds characterized by marked constriction along the midline of the vocal tract. These sounds include all the consonants; however, Chomsky and Halle did not consider /h/ /w/ and /j/ as consonantal—this text will treat them as consonantal.

Vocalic

Sounds produced with a relatively unobstructed oral cavity. Additionally, all vocalic sounds will be produced with voicing. All vowels are vocalic, but only the liquid consonants /l/ and /r/ have this feature.

Interrupted

Sounds produced by total blockage of the airflow at their point of constriction. The interrupted sounds include the stops /p b t d k g/ and the affricates /ʧ ʤ/.

Continuant

Sounds made with a continuation of the airflow through the oral cavity. Continuants include the glides /j w/, liquids /l r/, and fricatives /f v θ ð s z ʃ ʒ h/. Although it may seem that one is able to sustain production of the nasals, they are not considered continuants, because in their production, the airstream is directed through the nasal cavity rather than the oral cavity.

Strident

Sounds produced with high frequency turbulence causing them to be considered "noisier" than other consonants. Stridents include some fricatives /f v s z ʃ ʒ/ and both affricates /ʧ ʤ/.

Back

Sounds produced with a retracted tongue body beyond the neutral position of /ə/. The three velar phonemes are (+) for back /k g ŋ/. The glide /w/ is sometimes considered back, because it does have a velar production component. This text will not consider /w/ to be (+) back.

Anterior

The point of obstruction is located anterior to that of the palatal /ʃ/. The following phonemes are (+) anterior /w f v t d s z n l p b m Θ ð/.

Coronal

Sounds made with the tongue blade raised above the neutral position of /ə/. The coronal sounds include/ʒ ʃ ʤ ʧ ð θ s z t d l n j r/.

Lateral

Sound made by placing tip of the tongue against the alveolar ridge and lowering the midsection of the tongue, resulting in the airstream to flow over and around the sides of the tongue. There is only one lateral sound, the liquid /l/.

Rounded

Sounds produced with the lips pursed or protruded. Only two consonants are considered (+) rounded /r/ and /w/.

Labial

Sounds made with either or both lips. These sounds include the bilabials and the labio-dental phonemes. The (+) labial consonants are /p b m w f v r/.

Nasal

Sounds made with the velopharyngeal port open, so that the airstream is directed through the nasal cavity. There are three nasal sounds /m n ŋ/.

Voice

Sounds that are produced with vocal fold vibration. All the sonorants, including the nasals /m n ŋ/, the liquids /l r/, and the glides /w j/, are voiced. Additionally, the obstruent stops /b d g/, fricatives /v ð z ʒ/, and affricate /ʤ/ are voiced.

CONCLUSION

Classification schemes are a useful tool for SLPs to help organize and categorize sounds. They also aid in the understanding of the nature of the phonemes and their production features to use for practice. The more you practice, the more proficient you will become.

CHAPTER

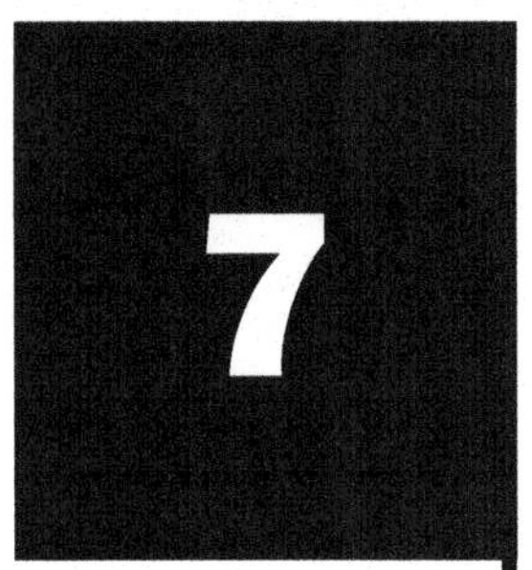

Chapter 6 introduced the characteristics and features that define the consonants and the ways in which consonant speech sounds can be classified. This chapter will focus on each consonant in detail with exercises presented to aid in transcription. Our discussion of the consonants will begin with the obstruents followed by the sonorants.

THE CONSONANTS

Obstruents

This major sound class describes sounds made with some degree of constriction within the vocal tract that impedes or completely obstructs the airflow (Ohde & Sharf, 1992). Obstruents include stops, fricatives, and affricates.

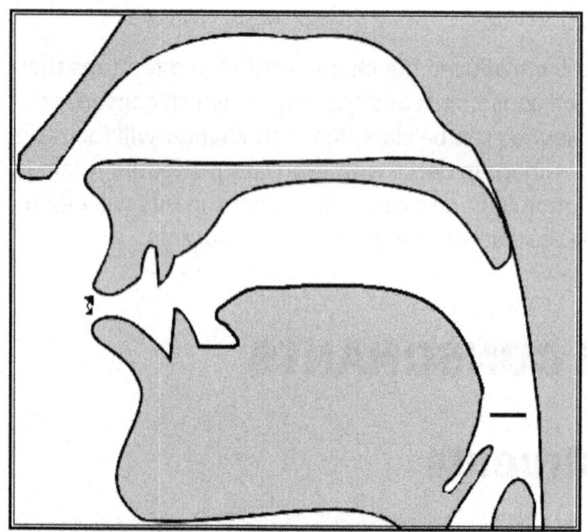

Fig. 7.1: P

Stops

/p/: Keyword *pay* /pe/

How it is made:

Airflow from the lungs is stopped at the point of the lips, which are firmly closed.

Velopharyngeal port is closed.

Vocal folds are abducted.

Lips part, releasing the airflow in an explosive manner.

Distinctive Features (Chomsky & Halle, 1968):

+: Obstruent, Consonantal, Interrupted, Anterior, Labial

-: Sonorant, Vocalic, Continuant, Strident, Back, Coronal, Rounded, Lateral, Nasal, Voice

Spellings beginning with the most common (Hanna et al., 1966):

p: pie

pp: happy

ph: shepherd

gh: hiccough

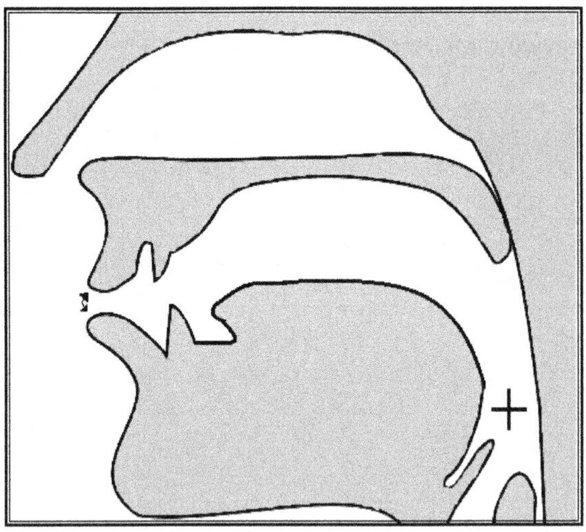

Fig. 7.2: B

/b/: Keyword *bye* /baɪ/

How it is made:

Lips are brought together.

Velopharyngeal port is closed.

Vocal folds are adducted.

Lips are parted, thus permitting the release of the sound.

Distinctive Features (Chomsky & Halle, 1968):

+: Obstruent, Consonantal, Interrupted, Anterior, Labial, Voice

-: Sonorant, Vocalic, Continuant, Strident, Back, Coronal, Rounded, Lateral, Nasal

Spellings beginning with the most common (Hanna et al., 1966):

b: boo

bb: gobble

pb: cupboard

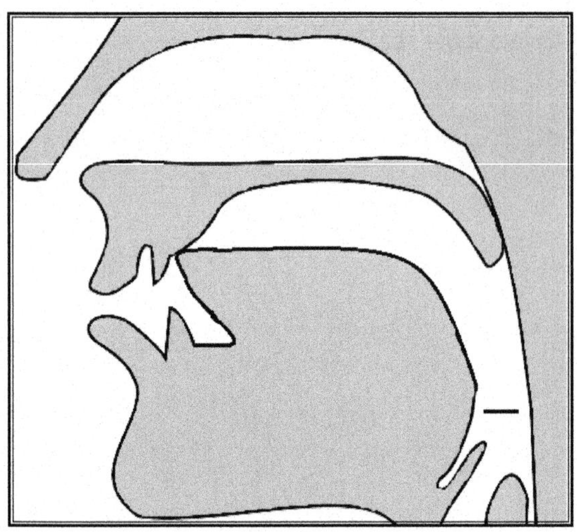

Fig. 7.3: T

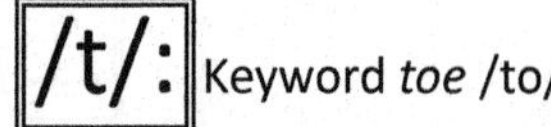

How it is made:

Tongue makes contact with the alveolar ridge, obstructing the airstream.

Velopharyngeal port is closed.

Vocal folds are abducted.

Tongue lowers, releasing the sound out of the mouth.

Distinctive Features (Chomsky & Halle, 1968):

+: Obstruent, Consonantal, Interrupted, Anterior, Coronal

-: Sonorant, Vocalic, Continuant, Strident, Back, Rounded, Lateral, Labial, Nasal, Voice

Spellings beginning with the most common (Hanna et al., 1966):

tt: bottle

bt: doubt

d: walked

pt: receipt

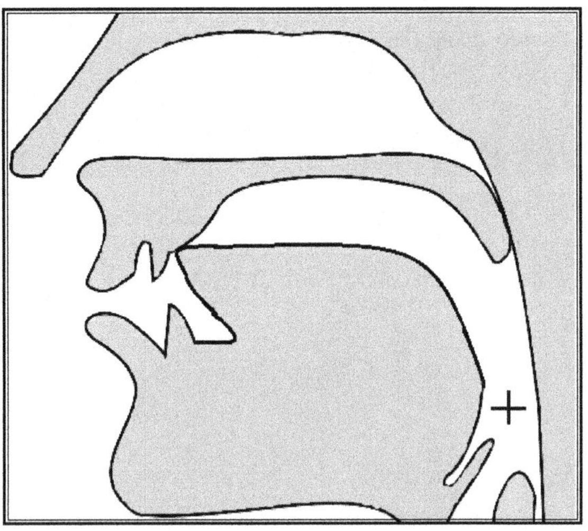

Fig. 7.4: D

/d/: Keyword *day* /de/

How it is made:

Tongue makes contact with the alveolar ridge, obstructing the airstream.

Velopharyngeal port is closed.

Vocal folds are adducted.

Tongue lowers, releasing the sound out of the mouth.

Distinctive Features (Chomsky & Halle, 1968):

+: Obstruent, Consonantal, Interrupted, Anterior, Coronal, Voice

-: Sonorant, Vocalic, Continuant, Strident, Back, Rounded, Lateral, Labial, Nasal

Spellings beginning with the most common (Hanna et al., 1966):

d: dew

dd: cuddle

ed: wanted

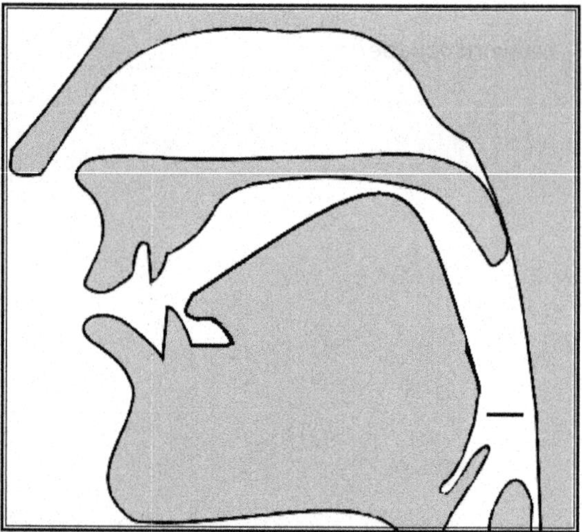

Fig. 7.5: K

/k/: Keyword *key* /ki/

How it is made:

Back of the tongue makes contact with the velum, obstructing the airstream.

Velopharyngeal port is closed.

Vocal folds are abducted.

Tongue lowers releasing the sound out of the mouth.

Distinctive Features (Chomsky & Halle, 1968):

+: Obstruent, Consonantal, Interrupted, Back

-: Sonorant, Vocalic, Continuant, Strident, Anterior, Coronal, Rounded, Lateral, Labial, Nasal, Voice

Spellings beginning with the most common (Hanna et al., 1966):

c: car

k: keep

ck: tack

cc: occur

ch: schedule

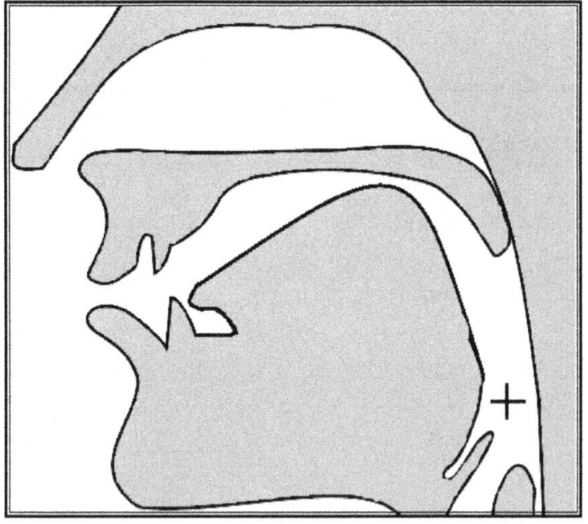

Fig. 7.6: G

/g/: Keyword *go* /go/

How it is made:

Back of the tongue makes contact with the velum, obstructing the airstream.

Velopharyngeal port is closed.

Vocal folds are adducted.

Tongue lowers, releasing the sound out of the mouth.

Distinctive Features (Chomsky & Halle, 1968):

+: Obstruent, Consonantal, Interrupted, Back, Voice

-: Sonorant, Vocalic, Continuant, Strident, Anterior, Coronal, Rounded, Lateral, Labial, Nasal

Spellings beginning with the most common (Hanna et al., 1966):

g: gate

gg: goggles

gh: gherkin

Exercise 7.1 Identify the following words:

1. /ʌpɚ/	upper	16. /pop/	pope
2. /bʌd/	bud	17. /pækt/	packed
3. /pʌp/	pup	18. /dip/	deep
4. /pɑp/	pop	19. /tep/	tape
5./pæd/	pad	20. /bip/	beep
6./kʌt/	cut	21. /gʌt/	gut
7./bæg/	bag	22. /tept/	taped
8./dɑkt/	docked	23. /detə/	data
9./totɛd/	totted	24. /pɪki/	picky
10./tæki/	tacky	25. /pɝki/	perky
11. /kot/	coat	26. /botɚ/	boater
12. /bɑbi/	bobby	27. /kæbi/	cabbie
13. /bʌtɚ/	butter	28. /ədæpt/	adapt
14. /kæt/	cat	29. /gaɪ/	guy
15. /daɪd/	died	30. /kʌp/	cup

Exercise 7.2 Transcribe the following words:

1. ape	/ep/	5. good	/gʊd/
2. peep	/pip/	6. tick	/tIk/
3. beat	/bit/	7. guppy	/gʌpi/
4. back	/bæk/	8. paperback	/pe.pɚbæk/

9. pucker /pʌkɚ/
10. dog /dag/
11. took /tʊk/
12. bigger /bɪgɚ/
13. dagger /dægɚ/
14. debate /dəbet/
15. attack /ətæk/
16. but /bʌt/
17. bed /bɛd/
18. pet /pɛt/
19. Abe /eb/
20. puppet /pʌpɪt/
21. cookie /kʊki/
22. doctor /dɑktɚ/
23. pack /pæk/
24. cape /kep/
25. taupe /top/
26. putt /pʌt/
27. bagboy /bægbɔɪ/
28. dirty /dɝti/
29. ticket /tɪkɪt/
30. toad /tod/

Exercise 7.3 Complete the Distinctive Feature Chart. Refer to Distinctive Features in Chapter 6 to check your answers:

Distinctive Feature: Stops

Stops	/p/	/b/	/t/	/d/	/k/	/g /
Obstruent	+	+	+	+	+	+
Sonorant	–	–	–	–	–	–
Consonantal	+	+	+	+	+	+

(*Continued*)

Vocalic	−	−	−	−	−	−
Continuant	−	−	−	−	−	−
Interrupted	+	+	+	+	+	+
Anterior	+	+	+	+	−	−
Back	−	−	−	−	+	+
Strident	−	−	−	−	−	−
Coronal	−	−	+	+	−	−
Lateral	−	−	−	−	−	−
Rounded	−	−	−	−	−	−
Labial	+	+	−	−	−	−
Nasal	−	−	−	−	−	−
Voice	−	+	−	+	−	+
Stops	/p/	/b/	/t/	/d/	/k/	/g/

Exercise 7.4 Complete the Stop Crossword Puzzle

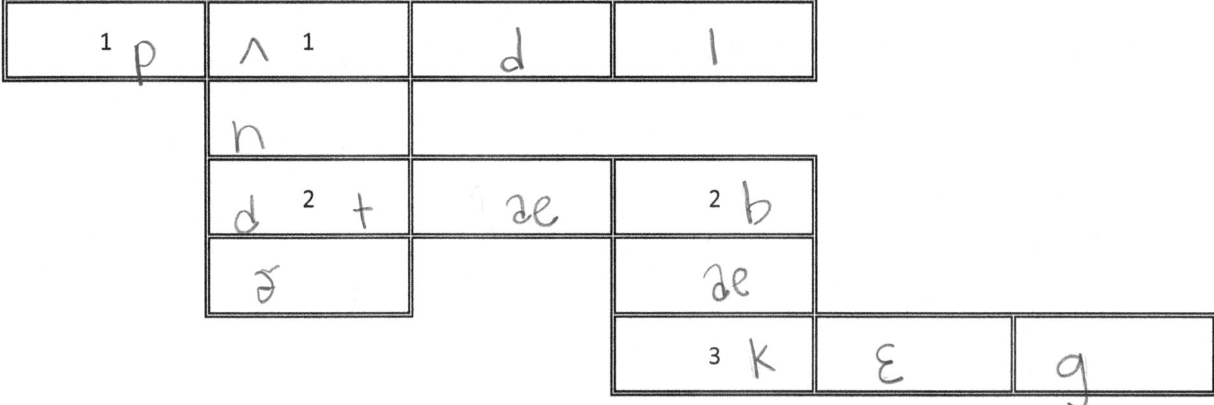

Down	Across
1. under	1. puddle
2. back	2. tab
	3. keg

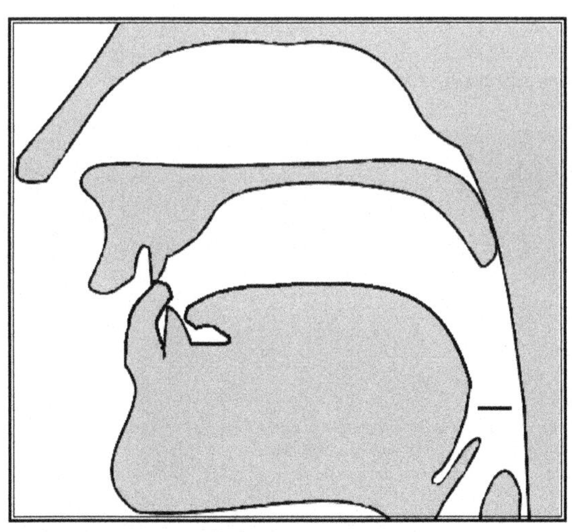

Fig. 7.7: F

Fricatives

/f/: Keyword *feet* /fit/

How it is made:

Edges of the upper central incisors come in contact with the lower lip.

Velopharyngeal port is closed.

(*Continued*)

Vocal folds are abducted.

Airflow is forced through the narrow constriction.

Distinctive Features (Chomsky & Halle, 1968):

+: Obstruent, Consonantal, Continuant, Anterior, Strident, Labial

-: Sonorant, Vocalic, Interrupted, , Back, Coronal, Lateral, Rounded, Nasal, Voice

Spellings beginning with the most common (Hanna et al., 1966):

f: fit

ph: photograph

ff: off

gh: rough

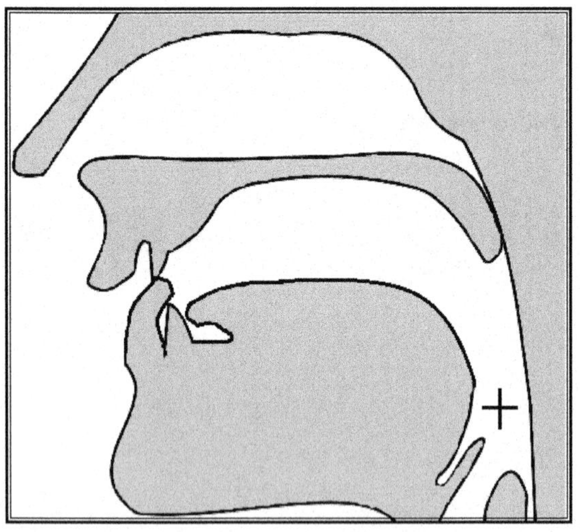

Fig. 7.8: V

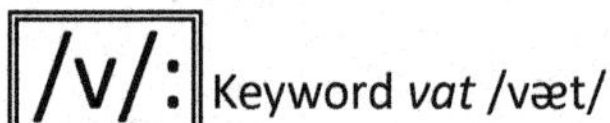

Keyword *vat* /væt/

How it is made:

Edges of the upper central incisors come in contact with the lower lip.

Velopharyngeal port is closed.

Vocal folds are adducted.

Airflow is forced through the narrow constriction.

Distinctive Features (Chomsky & Halle, 1968):

+: Obstruent, Consonantal, Continuant, Anterior, Strident, Labial, Voice

-: Sonorant, Vocalic, Interrupted, Back, Coronal, Lateral, Rounded, Nasal

Spellings beginning with the most common (Hanna et al., 1966):

v: vet

f: of

ph: Stephen

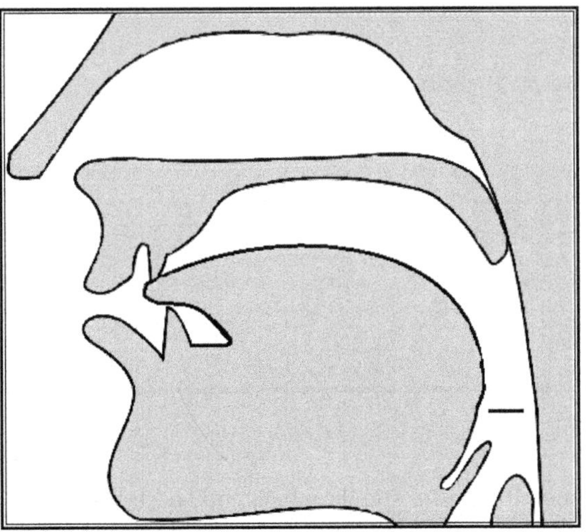

Fig. 7.9: TH - Voiceless

/θ/: Keyword *thaw* /θɔ/

How it is made:

Flattened tongue shifts forward and rests in the space between the teeth. Lips are slightly parted and neutral.

Velopharyngeal port is closed.

Vocal folds are abducted.

Airflow is forced through the narrow constriction.

Distinctive Features (Chomsky & Halle, 1968):

+: Obstruent, Consonantal, Continuant, Anterior, Coronal

-: Sonorant, Vocalic, Interrupted, Strident, Back, Rounded, Lateral, Labial, Nasal, Voice

Spellings beginning with the most common (Hanna et al., 1966):

th: theta

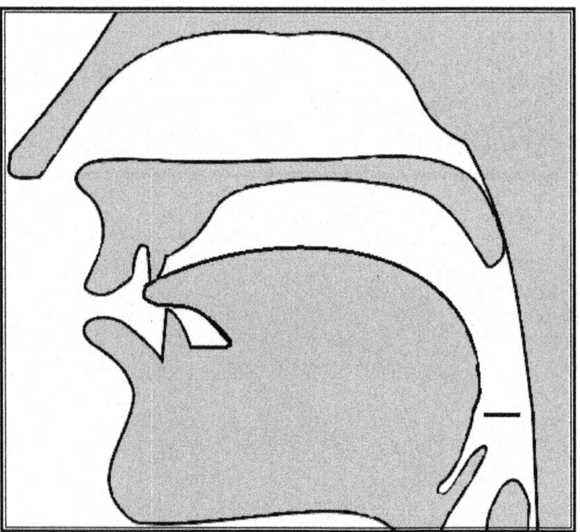

Fig. 7.10: TH – Voiced

/ð/: Keyword *these* /ðiz/

How it is made:

Flattened tongue shifts forward and rests in the space between the teeth. The lips are slightly parted and neutral.

Velopharyngeal port is closed.

Vocal folds are adducted.

Airflow is forced through the narrow constriction.

Distinctive Features (Chomsky & Halle, 1968):

+: Obstruent, Consonantal, Continuant, Anterior, Coronal, Voice

-: Sonorant, Vocalic, Interrupted, Strident, Back, Rounded, Lateral, Labial, Nasal

Spellings beginning with the most common (Hanna et al., 1966):

th: though

the: teethe

It can be very difficult to determine if a *"th"* sound is voiced or voiceless. As with anything, your ability to discriminate between /θ/ and /ð/ will come with practice. When completing the exercise that follows, it might be helpful to articulate the *"th"* sound apart from the rest of the word to see if it is produced with voicing or not. For example, say *"th-ank,"* to determine if voicing is present.

Prevocalic, Postvocalic, and Intervocalic *"th"*

Exercise 7.5 Circle whether the voicing of the two words is the same or different:

Words:		Voicing: Same or Different
1. thy	thigh	S (D)
2. bath	bathe	S (D)
3. thunder	thirsty	(S) D
4. these	thumb	S (D)
5. thin	third	(S) D
6. with	wither	S (D)
7. smooth	wreath	S (D)
8. breathe	breath	S (D)
9. soothe	south	S (D)
10. myth	mouth	(S) D

(Continued)

11. either	nothing	S (D)
12. leather	lethal	S (D)
13. sympathy	authentic	(S) D
14. gather	mother	(S) D
15. worthy	breathy	S (D)
16. farther	father	(S) D
17. teeth	teethe	S (D)

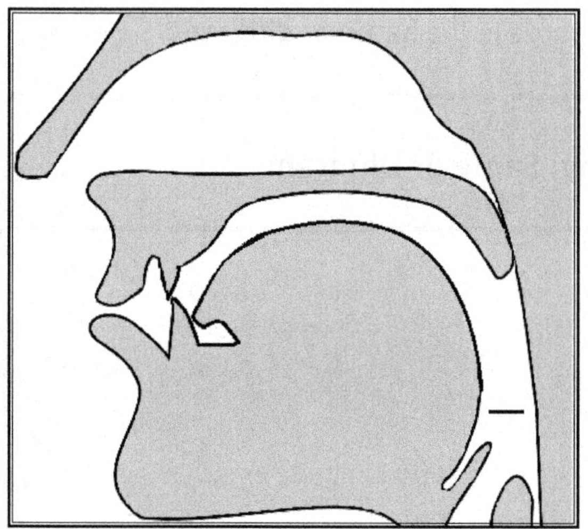

Fig. 7.11: S

/s/: Keyword *say* /se/

How it is made:

Grooved tongue approximates the alveolar ridge and makes contact with the ridge laterally. Lips are parted and neutral.

Velopharyngeal port is closed.

Vocal folds are abducted.

Airstream is directed through the groove in the tongue, creating turbulence.

Distinctive Features (Chomsky & Halle, 1968):

+: Obstruent, Consonantal, Continuant, Anterior, Strident, Coronal

-: Sonorant, Vocalic, Interrupted, Back, Rounded, Lateral, Nasal, Labial, Voice

Spellings beginning with the most common (Hanna et al., 1966):

s: sew

c: cease

ss: glass

sc: sciatica

sw: answer

z: glitz

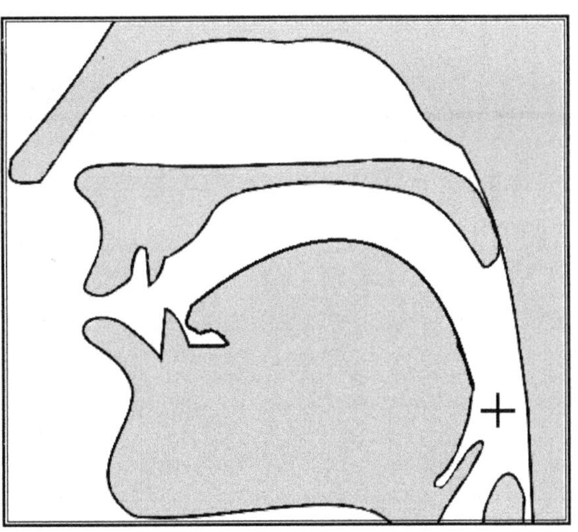

Fig. 7.12: Z

/z/: Keyword *zoo* /zu/

How it is made:

Grooved tongue approximates the alveolar ridge and makes contact with the ridge laterally. Lips are parted and neutral.

(*Continued*)

Velopharyngeal port is closed.

Vocal folds are adducted.

Airstream is directed through the groove in the tongue, creating turbulence.

Distinctive Features (Chomsky & Halle, 1968):

+: Obstruent, Consonantal, Continuant, Anterior, Strident, Coronal, Voice

-: Sonorant, Vocalic, Interrupted, Back, Rounded, Lateral, Labial, Nasal

Spellings beginning with the most common (Hanna et al., 1966):

s: paws

z: zipper

es: judges

ss: scissors

x: xylograph

zz: puzzle

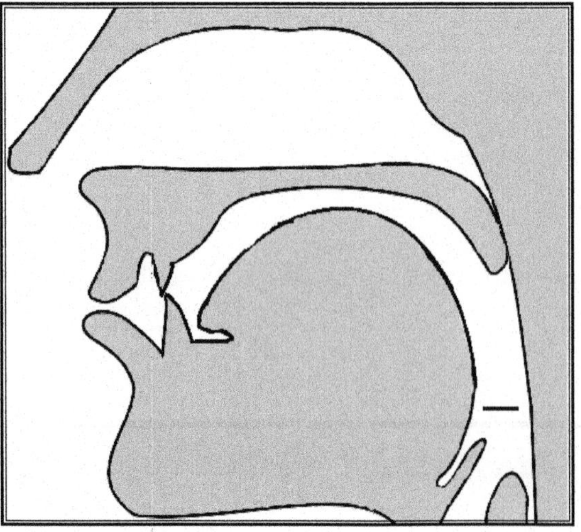

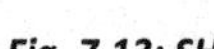

Fig. 7.13: SH

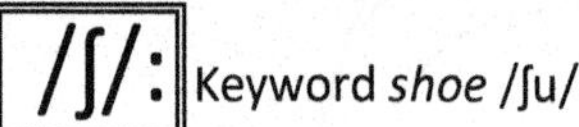

/ʃ/: Keyword *shoe* /ʃu/

How it is made:

Grooved tongue (broader groove than that of the /t/ and /d/) makes contact with the upper molars laterally. Lips are typically rounded and somewhat protruded.

Velopharyngeal port is closed.

Vocal folds are abducted.

Turbulence is created as the airstream passes against the hard palate, alveolar ridge, and teeth.

Distinctive Features (Chomsky & Halle, 1968):

+: Obstruent, Consonantal, Continuant, Strident, Coronal

-: Sonorant, Vocalic, Interrupted, Anterior, Back, Lateral, Rounded, Labial, Nasal, Voice

Spellings beginning with the most common (Hanna et al., 1966):

ti: fiction

sh: shop

ssi: permission

ch: Champagne

ci: social

s: sure

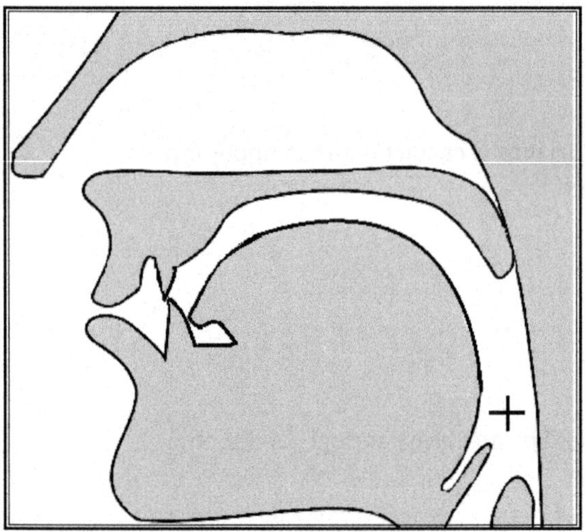

Fig. 7.14 ZH

/ʒ/: Keyword *leisure* /liʒɚ/

How it is made:

Grooved tongue (broader groove than that of the /t/ and /d/) makes contact with the upper molars, laterally. Lips are typically rounded and somewhat protruded.

Velopharyngeal port is closed.

Vocal folds are adducted.

Turbulence is created as the airstream passes against the hard palate, alveolar ridge, and teeth.

Distinctive Features (Chomsky & Halle, 1968):

+: Obstruent, Consonantal, Continuant, Strident, Coronal, Voice

-: Sonorant, Vocalic, Interrupted, Anterior, Back, Lateral, Rounded, Labial, Nasal

Spellings beginning with the most common (Hanna et al., 1966):

si: occasion

s: pleasure

z: azure

g: subterfuge

ti: equation

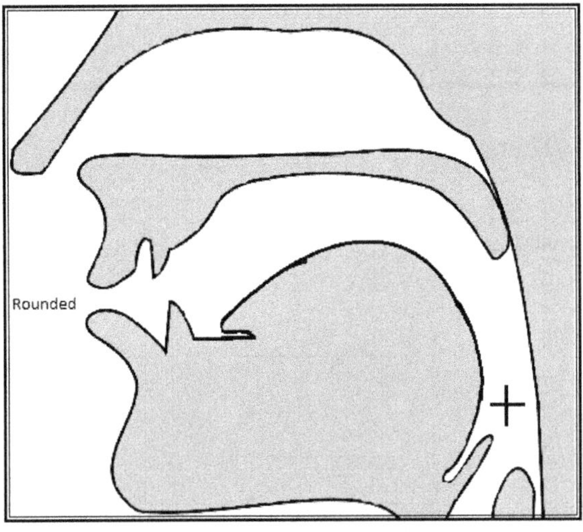

Fig. 7.15 H

/h/: Keyword *high* /haɪ/

How it is made:

Airflow is forced through a constriction created by the narrowing of the vocal folds. Tongue and lips are in position to produce the vowel that follows the /h/.

Velopharyngeal port is closed.

Vocal folds are abducted.

Distinctive Features (Chomsky & Halle, 1968):

+: Obstruent, Consonantal, Continuant

-: Sonorant, Vocalic, Interrupted, Strident, Anterior, Coronal, Lateral, Back, Rounded, Labial, Nasal, Voice

Spellings beginning with the most common (Hanna et al., 1966):

h: home

wh: whom

Exercise 7.6 Identify the following words:

1. /tuθ/	tooth	16. /ʃʊgɚ/	sugar
2. /sɪti/	city	17. /sɪzɚz/	scissors
3. /sʌpɚ/	supper	18. /ʃɑk/	shock
4. /fɪʃ/	fish	19. /sit/	seat
5. /kæʃ/	cash	20. /hæθ/	hath
6. /dɪʃɛz/	dishes	21. /kæst/	cast
7. /sɑk/	sock	22. /æʒɚ/	azure
8. /ʃʌks/	shucks	23. /hʌʃt/	hushed
9. /pæst/	past	24. /skɝt/	skirt
10. /fɪzd/	fizzed	25. /ʃaʊt/	shout
11. /ʃɝt/	shirt	26. /ðʌs/	thus
12. /huz/	who's	27. /vɔɪs/	voice
13. /bɑðɚ/	bother	28. /ʃɛd/	shed
14. /vaɪzɚ/	visor	29. /ʃu/	shoe
15. /ʃip/	sheep	30. /fɑks/	fox

Exercise 7.7 Transcribe the following words:

1. five	/faɪv/	16. zip	/zɪp/
2. tease	/tiz/	17. hers	/hɝz/
3. zoo	/zu/	18. eyes	/aɪz/
4. Bob's	/Babz/	19. zigzag	/zɪgzæg/
5. huff	/hʌf/	20. shaves	/ʃevz/
6. oars	/ɔrz/	21. hat	/hæt/
7. high	/haɪ/	22. tough	/tʌf/
8. thigh	/θaɪ/	23. thumb	/θʌm/
9. theft	/θɛft/	24. heft	/hɛft/
10. sad	/sæd/	25. veto	/vito/
11. vase	/ves/	26. have	/hæv/
12. thought	/θat/	27. these	/ðiz/
13. vote	/vot/	28. dashes	/dæʃɪz/
14. fate	/fet/	29. beige	/bedʒ/
15. soap	/sop/	30. cost	/kast/

Exercise 7.8 Complete the Distinctive Feature Charts. Refer to Distinctive Features in Chapter 6 to check your answers:

Distinctive Features: Fricatives

Fricatives	/f/	/v/	/θ/	/ð/	/s/	/z/	/ʃ/	/ʒ/	/h/
Obstruent	+	+	+	+	+	+	+	+	+
Sonorant	−	−	−	−	−	−	−	−	−
Consonantal	+	+	+	+	+	+	+	+	+
Vocalic	−	−	−	−	−	−	−	−	−
Continuant	+	+	+	+	+	+	+	+	+
Interrupted	−	−	−	−	−	−	−	−	−
Anterior	+	+	+	+	+	+	−	−	−
Back	−	−	−	−	−	−	−	−	−
Strident	+	+	−	−	+	+	+	+	−
Coronal	−	−	+	+	+	+	+	+	−
Lateral	−	−	−	−	−	−	−	−	−
Rounded	−	−	−	−	−	−	−	−	−
Labial	+	+	−	−	−	−	−	−	−
Nasal	−	−	−	−	−	−	−	−	−
Voice	−	+	−	+	−	+	−	+	−
Fricatives	/f/	/v/	/θ/	/ð/	/s/	/z/	/ʃ/	/ʒ/	/h/

Exercise 7.9 Identify what is wrong with the following words. If the word is correct, write "ok"; if the word is incorrect, correct it:

1. push/pʊsh/ ________	6. /of/ /ʌf/ ________
2. back/bæck/ ________	7. off/ɑff/ ________
3. pop/pop/ ________	8. /ship//ʃɪp/ ________
4. soft/sɑft/ ________	9. /host//host/ ________
5. sheep/ʃeep/ ________	10. twos/tus/ ________

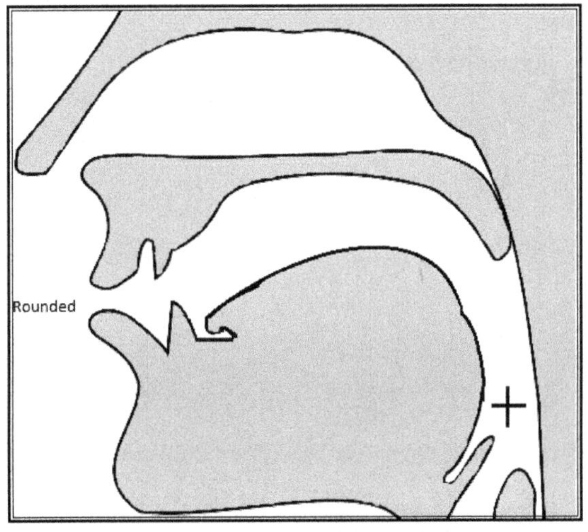

Fig. 7.16 CH

Affricates

/ʧ/: Keyword *Chip* /ʧɪp/

How it is made:

Tongue moves forward and makes contact with the alveolar ridge; tongue then releases and retracts, forming a channel.

Velopharyngeal port is closed.

Vocal folds are abducted.

Airstream is briefly blocked at the alveolar ridge, but on release, turbulence is created as the tongue flattens along the palate.

(*Continued*)

Distinctive Features (Chomsky & Halle, 1968):

+: Obstruent, Consonantal, Interrupted, Strident, Coronal

-: Sonorant, Vocalic, Continuant, Anterior, Back, Rounded, Lateral, Labial, Nasal, Voice

Spellings beginning with the most common (Hanna et al., 1966):

ch: chocolate

t: mature

tch: itch

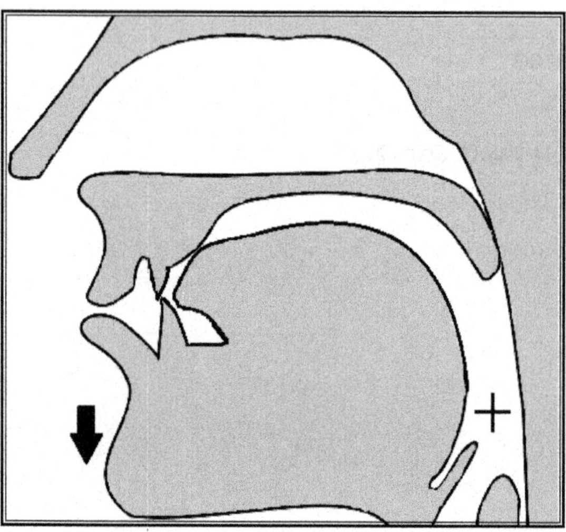

Fig. 7.17 DG

/ʤ/: Keyword *judge* /ʤʌʤ/

How it is made:

Tongue moves forward and makes contact with the alveolar ridge; tongue then releases and retracts, forming a channel.

Velopharyngeal port is closed.

Vocal folds are adducted.

Airstream is briefly blocked at the alveolar ridge, but on release, turbulence is created as the tongue flattens along the palate.

Distinctive Features (Chomsky & Halle, 1968):

+: Obstruent, Consonantal, Interrupted, Strident, Coronal, Voice

-: Sonorant, Vocalic, Continuant, Anterior, Back, Rounded, Lateral, Labial, Nasal

Spellings beginning with the most common (Hanna et al., 1966):

g: germ

j: juice

dg: judge

d: educator

di: soldier

dj: adjust

gg: exaggerate

gi: legion

Exercise 7.10 Identify the following words:

1. / ʤaʊst/	joust	11. /ʤɛst/	jest
2. /ʤe/	jay	12. /fʌʤ/	fudge
3. /ʤɛsʧɚ/	gesture	13. /ʤʌg/	jug
4. /səʤɛst/	suggest	14. /hæʧɛz/	hatches
5. /bʊʧɚ/	butcher	15. /bɑʧɛz/	batches
6. /fiʧɚ/	feature	16. /əbʤɛkt/	object
7. /ʤæk/	jack	17. /fɛʧɛz/	fetches
8. /poʧɛz/	poaches	18. /kɛʧəp/	ketchup
9. /tʌʧɛz/	touches	19. /dʌʧɛz/	duchess
10. /ʤɛt/	jet	20. /piʧɛz/	peaches

Exercise 7.11 Transcribe the following words:

1. chuck	/tʃʌk/	11. choppy	/tʃapi/
2. choke	/tʃok/	12. lecture	/lɛktʃɚ/
3. picture	/pɪktʃɚ/	13. chug	/tʃʌg/
4. church	/tʃɝtʃ/	14. jig	/dʒɪg/
5. jeer	/dʒɛr/	15. choose	/tʃuz/
6. jiffy	/dʒɪfi/	16. gin	/dʒɪn/
7. chubby	/tʃʌbi/	17. jade	/dʒed/
8. gipsy	/dʒɪpsi/	18. pasture	/pæstʃɚ/
9. jigsaw	/dʒɪgsɔ/	19. jitters	/dʒɪtɚz/
10. chew	/tʃu/	20. chose	/tʃoz/

Exercise 7.12 Complete the Distinctive Feature Charts. Refer to Distinctive Features in Chapter 6 to check your answers.

Affricates	/tʃ/	/dʒ/
Obstruent	+	+
Sonorant	–	–
Consonantal	+	+

Vocalic	−	−
Continuant	−	−
Interrupted	+	+
Anterior	−	−
Back	−	−
Strident	+	+
Coronal	+	+
Lateral	−	−
Rounded	−	−
Labial	−	−
Nasal	−	−
Voice	−	+
Affricates	/tʃ/	/dʒ/

Obstruents	/p/	/b/	/t/	/d/	/k/	/g/	/f/	/v/	/θ/	/ð/	/s/	/z/	/ʃ/	/ʒ/	/h/	/ʧ/	/ʤ/
Obstruent	+	+	+	+	+	+	+	+	+	+	+	+	+	+		+	+
Sonorant	−	−	−	−	−	−	−	−	−	−	−	−	−	−	−	−	−
Consonantal	+	+	+	+	+	+	+	+	+	+	+	+	+	+	+	+	+
Vocalic	−	−	−	−	−	−	−	−	−	−	−	−	−	−	−	−	−
Continuant	−	−	−	−	−	−	+	+	+	+	+	+	+	+	+	−	−
Interrupted	+	+	+	+	+	+	−	−	−	−	−	−	−	−	−	+	+
Anterior	+	+	+	+	−	−	+	+	+	+	+	+	−	−	−	−	−
Back	−	−	−	−	+	+	−	−	−	−	−	−	−	−	−	−	−
Strident	−	−	−	−	−	−	+	+	−	−	+	+	+	+	−	+	+
Coronal	−	−	+	+	−	−	−	−	+	+	+	+	+	+	−	+	+
Lateral	−	−	−	−	−	−	−	−	−	−	−	−	−	−	−	−	−
Rounded	−	−	+	−	−	−	−	−	−	−	−	−	−	−	−	−	−
Labial	+	+	−	−	−	−	+	+	−	−	−	−	−	−	−	−	−
Nasal	−	−	−	−	−	−	−	−	−	−	−	−	−	−	−	−	−
Voice	−	+	−	+	−	+	−	+	−	+	−	+	−	+	−	−	+
Obstruents	/p/	/b/	/t/	/d/	/k/	/g/	/f/	/v/	/θ/	/ð/	/s/	/z/	/ʃ/	/ʒ/	/h/	/ʧ/	/ʤ/

Exercise 7. 13 Complete the Affricate Crossword Puzzle:

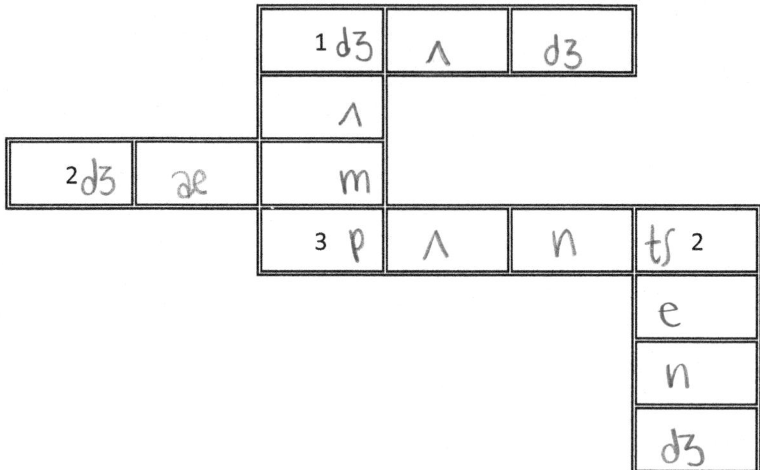

Down	**Across**
1. jump	1. judge
2. change	2. jam
	3. punch

Sonorants

This major sound class describes all vowels and the consonants that are produced with a relatively unobstructed vocal tract. Sonorant consonants are characterized by alterations of resonating cavities, have a vowel-like quality, and are always voiced (Ohde & Sharf, 1992). There are three different groupings of sonorant consonants: glides, liquids, and nasals.

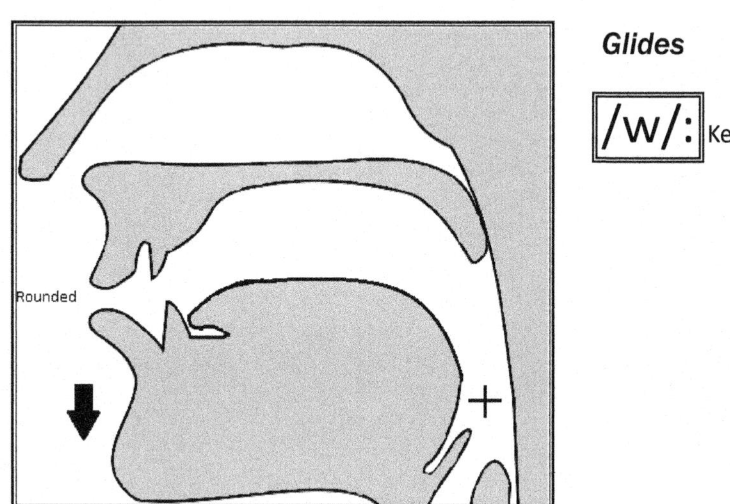

Fig. 7.18 W

Glides

/w/: Keyword *way* /we/

How it is made:

Lips round as the back of the tongue approximates the velum.

Velopharyngeal port is closed.

Vocal folds are adducted.

Lips sustain a gliding movement into the vowel that follows the /w/.

Distinctive Features (Chomsky & Halle, 1968):

+: Sonorant, Vocalic, Continuant, Anterior, Rounded, Labial, Voice

-: Obstruent, Consonantal, Interrupted, Strident, Back, Coronal, Lateral, Nasal

Spellings beginning with the most common (Hanna et al., 1966):

w: win

o: one

wh: when

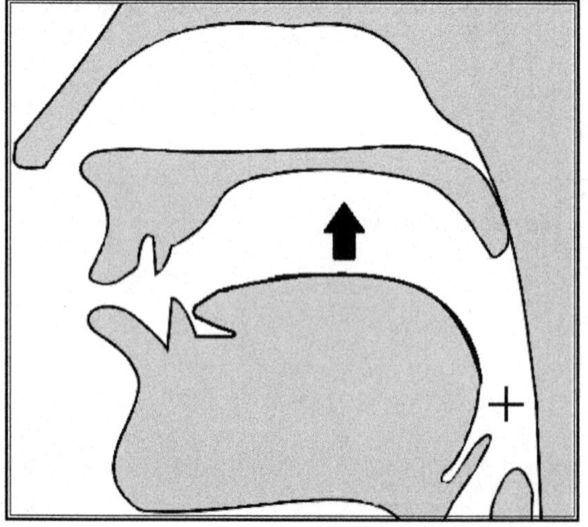

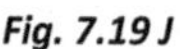

Fig. 7.19 J

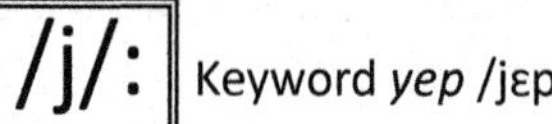

/j/: Keyword *yep* /jɛp/

How it is made:

Tongue is in a high front position similar to that for production of the vowel /i/ and is somewhat flattened toward the palate.

Velopharyngeal port is closed.

Vocal folds are adducted.

Lips and tongue glide into the movement needed to produce the vowel that follows.

Distinctive Features (Chomsky & Halle, 1968):

+: Sonorant, Vocalic, Continuant, Coronal, Rounded, Labial, Voice

-: Obstruent, Consonantal, Interrupted, Strident, Back, Anterior, Lateral, Nasal

Spellings beginning with the most common (Hanna et al., 1966):

i: scallion

y: yuck

ll: rebellion

Exercise 7.14 Transcribe the following words:

1. wood	/wʊd/	11. use	/juz/
2. wake	/wek/	12. wed	/wɛd/
3. wave	/wev/	13. weave	/wiv/
4. witch	/wɪtʃ/	14. whack	/wæk/
5. wig	/wɪg/	15. wick	/wɪk/
6. word	/wɝd/	16. yet	/jɛt/
7. wish	/wɪʃ/	17. wet	/wɛt/
8. way	/we/	18. yoke	/jok/
9. wait	/wet/	19. yea	/je/
10. yeah	/jæ/	20. wow	/waʊ/

Exercise 7.15 Complete the Distinctive Feature Charts. Refer to Distinctive Features in Chapter 6 to check your answers:

Glides	/w/	/j/
Obstruent	−	−
Sonorant	+	+
Consonantal	−	−
Vocalic	+	+
Continuant	+	+
Interrupted	−	−
Anterior	+	−
Back	−	−
Strident	−	−
Coronal	−	+
Lateral	−	−
Rounded	+	+
Labial	+	+
Nasal	−	−
Voice	+	+
Glides	/w/	/j/

Exercise 7.16 Complete the Glide Crossword Puzzle:

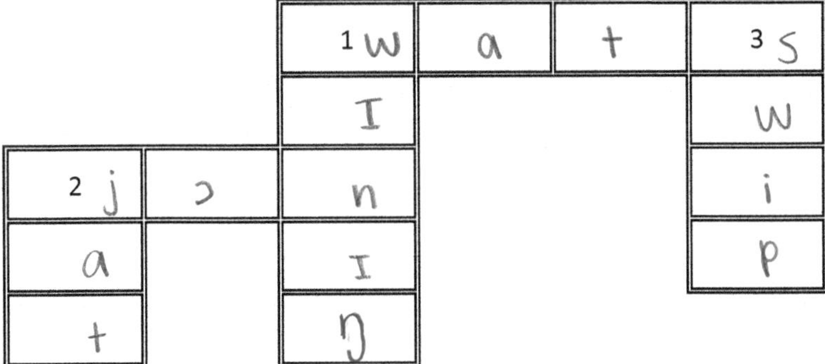

Down
1. winning
2. yacht
3. sweep

Across
1. watts
2. yawn

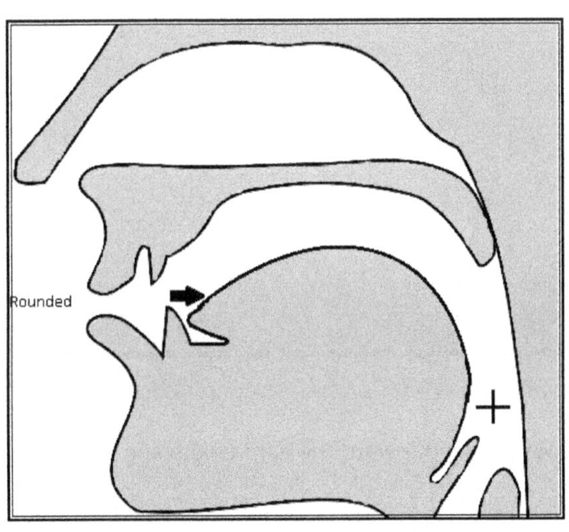

Fig. 7.20 L

Liquids

/l/: Keyword *lay* /le/

How it is made:

Tongue makes contact with the alveolar ridge. Lips are apart and in a neutral position.

Velopharyngeal port is closed.

Vocal folds are adducted.

Air flows over the sides of tongue.

(*Continued*)

Distinctive Features (Chomsky & Halle, 1968):

+: Sonorant, Consonantal, Vocalic, Continuant, Anterior, Coronal, Lateral, Voice

-: Obstruent, Interrupted, Strident, Back, Rounded, Labial, Nasal

Spellings beginning with the most common (Hanna et al., 1966):

l: like

ll: dull

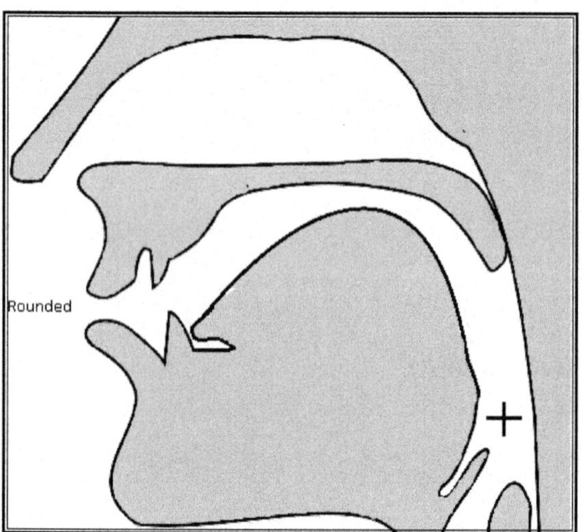

Fig. 7.21 R

/r/: Keyword *ray* /re/

How it is made:

Tongue root is retracted into the pharynx, and the tongue body is raised toward the hard palate and retracted or tightly "bunched." Lips are slightly rounded.

Velopharyngeal port is closed.

Vocal folds are adducted.

Distinctive Features (Chomsky & Halle, 1968):

+: Sonorant, Consonantal, Vocalic, Continuant, Coronal, Rounded, Labial, Voice

-: Obstruent, Interrupted, Anterior, Strident, Back, Lateral, Nasal

Spellings beginning with the most common (Hanna et al., 1966):

r: rat

rr: carrot

wr: wrong

Exercise 7.17 Identify the following words:

1. /lɑbstɚ/	lobster	6. /ple/	play
2. /stɑrz/	stars	7. /pɪlo/	pillow
3. /lɪpstɪk/	lipstick	8. /pɝLz/	pearls
4. /kənstrʌkt/	construct	9. /rezɔrbæks/	razorbacks
5. /dɛltə/	delta	10. /litʃ/	leech

Exercise 7.18 Transcribe the following words:

1. laugh	/læf/	11. lurk	/lɝk/
2. girl	/gɝl/	12. warrior	/wɔriɚ/
3. circles	/sɝklɛz/	13. Jello	/dʒɛlo/
4. reword	/riwɝd/	14. repute	/ripjut/
5. flirtatious	/flɚteʃəs/	15. wrath	/ræθ/
6. reward	/riwɔrd/	16. loop	/lup/
7. lazy	/lezi/	17. bellow	/bɛlo/
8. allow	/əlaʊ/	18. leap	/lip/
9. legalize	/ligəlaɪz/	19. robin	/rabɪn/
10. Rick	/rɪk/	20. relish	/rɛlɪʃ/

Exercise 7.19 Complete the Distinctive Feature Charts. Refer to Distinctive Features in Chapter 6 to check your answers:

Distinctive Features: Liquids

Liquids	/l/	/r/
Obstruent	–	–
Sonorant	+	+
Consonantal	+	+
Vocalic	+	+
Continuant	+	+
Interrupted	–	–
Anterior	+	–
Back	–	–
Strident	–	–
Coronal	+	+
Lateral	+	–
Rounded	–	+
Labial	–	+
Nasal	–	–
Voice	+	+
Liquids	/l/	/r/

Exercise 7.20 Complete the Liquid Crossword Puzzle:

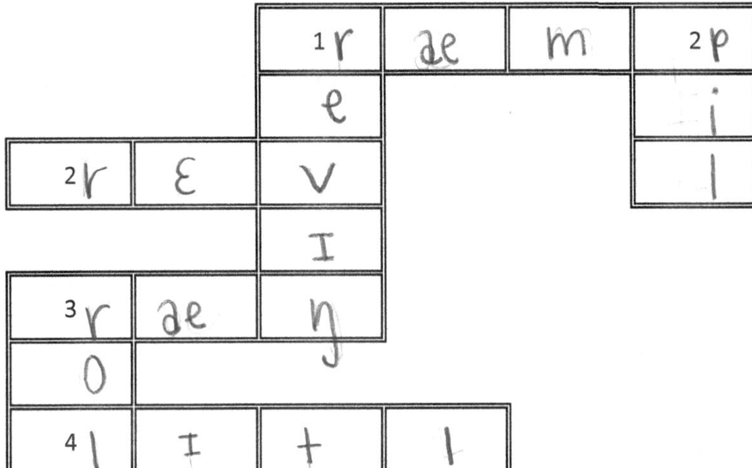

Down
1. raving
2. peel
3. roll

Across
1. ramp
2. rev
3. rang
4. little

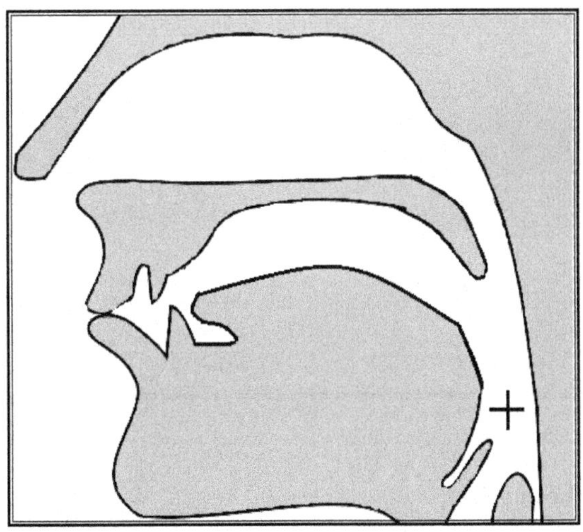

Fig. 7.22 M

Nasals

/m/: Keyword *may* /me/

How it is made:

Lips are brought together obstructing the airstream.

Velopharyngeal port is open.

Vocal folds are adducted.

(*Continued*)

Voiced airflow and acoustic vibrations continually flow into the nasal cavity and out the nose.

Distinctive Features (Chomsky & Halle, 1968):

+: Sonorant, Vocalic, Anterior, Labial, Nasal, Voice

-: Obstruent, Consonantal, Interrupted, Continuant, Strident, Back, Coronal, Rounded, Lateral

Spellings beginning with the most common (Hanna et al., 1966):

m: mom

mm: commentary

lm: palm

mb: comb

mn: hymn

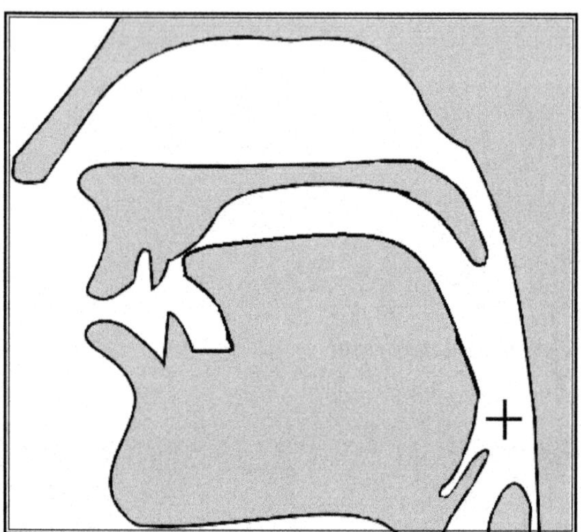

Fig. 7.23 N

/n/: Keyword *none* /nʌn/

How it is made:

Tongue makes contact with the alveolar ridge, obstructing the airstream.

Velopharyngeal port is open.

Vocal folds are adducted.

Voiced airflow and acoustic vibrations continually flow into the nasal cavity and out the nose.

Distinctive Features (Chomsky & Halle, 1968):

+: Sonorant, Vocalic, Anterior, Coronal, Nasal, Voice

-: Obstruent, Consonantal, Interrupted, Continuant, Strident, Back, Lateral, Rounded, Labial

Spellings beginning with the most common (Hanna et al., 1966):

n: now

gn: gnash

kn: knot

nn: winner

pn: pneumatic

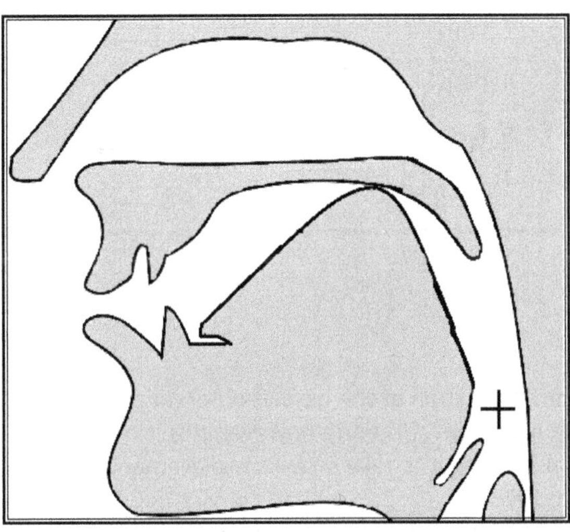

Fig. 7.24 ING

/ŋ/: Keyword *sing* /sɪŋ/

How it is made:

Back of the tongue makes contact with the velum, obstructing the airstream.

Velopharyngeal port is open.

Vocal folds are adducted.

Voiced airflow and acoustic vibrations continually flow into the nasal cavity and out the nose.

Distinctive Features (Chomsky & Halle, 1968):

+: Sonorant, Vocalic, Back, Nasal, Voice

-: Obstruent, Consonantal, Interrupted, Continuant, Strident, Anterior, Coronal, Lateral, Rounded, Labial

Spellings beginning with the most common (Hanna et al., 1966):

ng: song

n: pink

nd: handkerchief

Transcribing nasals + /æ/

Man vs. *Cat*: You might be surprised to find that *man* and *cat* contain the same vowel /æ/. The /æ/ sounds different in the word *man*, because it is nasalized due to the influence of the surrounding nasal consonants. According to Van Riper and Smith (1979), there are three vowels that are particularly influenced by nasality: /æ/, /ɛ/, and /i/.

Exercise 7.21 Complete the following exercises, which are designed to help with the transcription of words containing /æ/:

1. Santa	/saentə/	6. pang	/paeŋ/
2. panda	/paendə/	7. pansy	/paenzi/
3. amber	/aembɚ/	8. dam	/daem/
4. Tampa	/taempə/	9. tan	/taen/
5. panic	/paenɪk/	10. family	/faeməli/

Transcribing *nk*

Bank and Band: Although *bank* and *band* are spelled similarly, the articulation of the nasal is different due to the influence of coarticulation. For example, the word *band* is pronounced *ban+d* [bænd]; however, this is not true for *bank*, because the velar placement of the /k/ influences the nasal, causing it to take on a velar placement, as well. Therefore, the word *bank* becomes [bæŋk] (Van Riper and Smith, 1979).

Exercise 7.22 Complete the following exercises, which are designed to help with the transcription of words containing *nk*:

1. prank	/praeŋk/	11. pink	/pɪŋk/
2. sank	/saeŋk/	12. rank	/raeŋk/
3. drank	/draeŋk/	13. tank	/taeŋk/
4. thank	/θaeŋk/	14. ink	/ɪŋk/
5. rink	/rɪŋk/	15. think	/θɪŋk/
6. link	/lɪŋk/	16. oink	/ɔɪŋk/
7. mink	/mɪŋk/	17. drink	/drɪŋk/
8. blank	/blaeŋk/	18. wink	/wɪŋk/
9. cufflink	/kʌfliŋk/	19. Hank	/haeŋk/
10. dank	/daeŋk/	20. shrink	/ʃrɪŋk/

Exercise 7.23 Identify the following words:

1. /mædi/	maddy	6. /keli/	Kaley
2. /grɛʧɛn/	Gretchen	7. /ɛli/	Ellie
3. /səmænθə/	samantha	8. /traɪdɛnt/	trident
4. /dɑLfɪn/	dolphin	9. /paɪntri/	pine tree
5. /gemkɑks/	gamecocks	10. /krɛsɛnt/	crescent

Exercise 7.24 Complete the Distinctive Feature Charts. Refer to Distinctive Features in Chapter 6 to check your answer:

Distinctive Features: Nasals

Nasals	/m/	/n/	/ŋ/
Obstruent	–	–	–
Sonorant	+	+	+
Consonantal	–	–	–
Vocalic	+	+	+
Continuant	–	–	–
Interrupted	–	–	–
Anterior	+	+	–
Back	–	–	+
Strident	–	–	–
Coronal	–	+	–

(Continued)

Lateral	−	−	−
Rounded	−	−	−
Labial	+	−	−
Nasal	+	+	+
Voice	+	+	+
Nasals	/m/	/n/	/ŋ/

Distinctive Features: Sonorants

Sonorants	/w/	/j/	/l/	/r/	/m/	/n/	/ŋ/
Obstruent	−	−	−	−	−	−	−
Sonorant	+	+	+	+	+	+	+
Consonantal	−	−	+	+	−	−	−
Vocalic	+	+	+	+	+	+	+
Continuant	+	+	+	+	−	−	−
Interrupted	−	−	−	−	−	−	−
Anterior	+	−	+	−	+	+	−
Back	−	−	−	−	−	−	+
Strident	−	−	−	−	−	+	−

Coronal	−	+	+	+	−	+	−
Lateral	−	−	+	+	−	−	−
Rounded	+	+	−	+	−	−	−
Labial	+	+	−	+	+	−	−
Nasal	−	−	−	−	+	+	+
Voice	+	+	+	+	+	+	+
Sonorants	/w/	/j/	/l/	/r/	/m/	/n/	/ŋ/

Exercise 7.25 Complete the Nasal Crossword Puzzle:

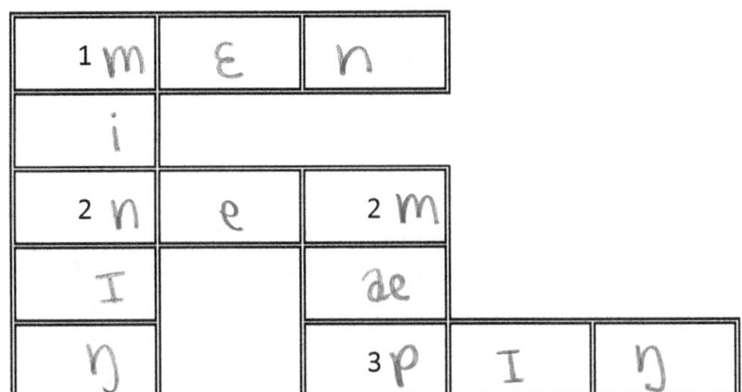

Down

1. meaning

2. map

Across

1. men

2. name

3. ping

The next exercises are designed to help you "put it all together."

Exercise 7.26 Circle the feature(s) that the phonemes have in common:

Manner- Place- Voice

1. /ʃ ŋ/	M P V	16. /p n/	M P V
2. /ʧ ʒ/	M P V	17. /j r/	M P V
3. /p n/	M P V	18. /r v/	M P V
4. /m b/	M P V	19. /k n/	M P V
5. /s l/	M P V	20. /k v/	M P V
6. /ʒ ʤ/	M P V	21. /h t/	M P V
7. /m n/	M P V	22. /t f/	M P V
8. /ʃ t/	M P V	23. /r ʃ/	M P V
9. /w j/	M P V	24. /l r/	M P V
10. /s n/	M P V	25. /v h/	M P V
11. /d g/	M P V	26. /j k/	M P V
12. /m g/	M P V	27. /f v/	M P V
13. /θ ð/	M P V	28. /n ʤ/	M P V
14. /ʃ ʧ/	M P V	29. /ʧ j/	M P V
15. /ʧ ʤ/	M P V	30. /g l/	M P V

Exercise 7.27 Change the listed feature(s) for the onset (phoneme in the initial position) of each word to create a minimal pair. Be sure to use the International Phonetic Alphabet (IPA):

Manner- Place- Voice

1. mast	M V	/pæst/
2. care	M P	/ʃɛr/
3. take	P	/kek/
4. pan	M V	/mæn/
5. band	M P	/lænd/
6. date	M P V	/fet/
7. sell	M	/tɛl/

8. hen	M P	/tɛn/
9. met	M	/bɛt/
10. chin	M P	/pɪn/
11. king	M P	/θɪŋ/
12. kit	P	/pɪt/
13. hoe	M P	/to/
14. might	P	/naɪt/
15. shut	P	/hʌt/
16. phone	P V	/zon/
17. bite	M P V	/faɪt/
18. rich	M P	/mɪtʃ/
19. Dutch	M P	/mʌtʃ/
20. dam	M V	/sæm/

Exercise 7.28 Identify what is wrong with the following words. If a word is transcribed incorrectly, correctly transcribe it. If a word is transcribed correctly, write "okay."

1. bigger	[bɪgɚ]	/bɪgɚ/
2. shut	[shʌt]	/ʃʌt/
3. bake	[bek]	ok
4. pepper	[pɛppɚ]	/pɛpɚ/
5. bother	[bɑθɚ]	/bɑðɚ/
6. bird	[bɪrd]	/bɝd/
7. black	[blæck]	/blæk/
8. panther	[pænthɚ]	/pænθɚ/
9. sink	[sɪnk]	/sɪŋk/
10. Dutch	[dʌttʃ]	/dʌtʃ/
11. king	[kɪŋ]	ok
12. bomb	[bɑmb]	/bɑm/
13. stow	[stow]	/sto/

(*Continued*)

14. might	[maɪt]	Ok
15. shop	[ʃɑp]]	Ok
16. phone	[fone]	/fon/
17. bite	[baɪte]	/baɪt/
18. case	[cese]	/kes/
19. supper	[sʌppɚ]	/sʌpɚ/
20. box	[bɑx]	/baks/
21. juice	[jus]	/dʒus/
22. pegs	[pɛgs]	/pɛgz/
23. wrong	[wrɔŋ]	/rɔŋ/
24. hope	[hope]	/hop/
25. picked	[pɪkɛd]	/pɪkt/

CONCLUSION

Vowels give our utterances power, while consonants provide the intelligibility. Although focusing on how words sound, rather than how they are spelled can be tricky, transcription will become easier with lots of practice, and you will become more proficient. Give it time, and before long, you will become a skilled transcriber.

CHAPTER

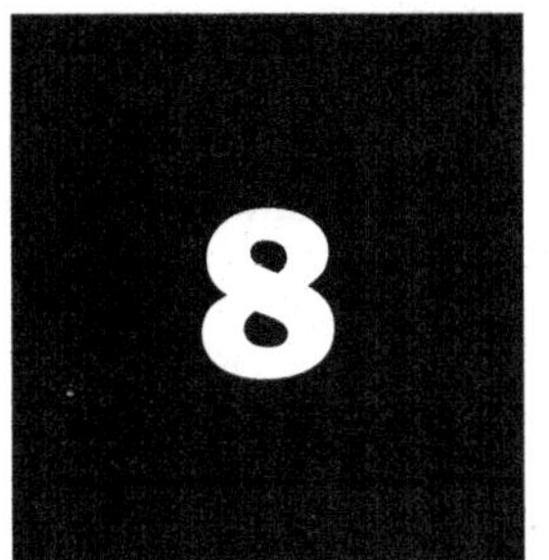

Producing language is a dynamic human behavior consisting of rules. An understanding of the rules for how we put sounds together to form words is vital to the speech-language pathologist (SLP) in the effective evaluation and treatment of speech sound disorders. Edwards and Shriberg (1983) outlined four areas of phonological knowledge that will be examined in this chapter. The first area is the understanding of the contrastive phonemes of a language. Previous chapters have introduced the symbols representing the speech sounds of English. Additionally, many exercises have been presented to assist you in using phonetic symbols (the International Phonetic Alphabet (IPA)) to transcribe words. You have also learned to classify phonemes according to their characteristics and features. However, words are not articulated one at a time, and phonemes are not produced in an invariant state. For this reason, Edwards and Shriberg suggested that acceptable allophonic sound variation is a parameter of our sound system that must also be examined; thus rules encompassing allophonic variations will be presented in this chapter. The third area of phonetic study addressed by Edwards and Shriberg was the permissible combination of sounds within languages, known as the study of phonotactics. This chapter will address the phontactic rules of English as summarized by Peña-Brooks and Hegde (2000). Lastly, morphophonemic adjustments are the final area of sound system study suggested by Edwards and Shriberg that will be presented. Morphophonemics refers to the sound alterations that result from certain morphological environments (O'Grady, Archibald, Aronoff & Rees-Miller, 2001). Morphophonemic rules as outlined by Peña-Brooks and Hegde (2000) are discussed below.

TRANSCRIBING CONNECTED SPEECH

It is estimated that 270 words are uttered per minute during conversational speech (Shipley and McAfee, 1998). When words are spoken in strings while conversing, this is referred to as "connected speech." Our articulators must make adjustments to meet the demands of rapidly moving from phoneme to phoneme. When speech is connected, the phonemes will change producing allophonic variations (Kent, 1998). Allophones and the differences between phonetic (narrow) and phonemic (broad) transcription were introduced in Chapter 2, and this chapter will address narrow transcription, which details speech as it is actually spoken, in connected utterances. The remaining chapters of this text will deal with the different applications of phonetic transcription. Recall that phonetic or "narrow" transcription documents the speech of an individual speaker. Phonetic transcription utilizes diacritical markings that are crucial for the description of speech variances, particularly disordered or different articulations. Sounds within a phonetic context influence one another, so in order to produce phonemes as rapidly and efficiently as possible, **accommodation**, the adjustments and adaptation of speech sounds (MacKay 1987), occurs. There are two types of accommodation, **assimilation** and **coarticulation**.

COARTICULATION AND ASSIMILATION

The complex adjustments made by our speech organs during connected speech are known as **coarticulation**. **Assimilation** is a coarticulatory process in which the sound alteration is so extensive that an audible change is noticed—the sound affected will take on perceptual qualities of an adjacent sound. Assimilation will result in major changes that can be perceived by the listener. According to Van Riper & Smith (1979), assimilation occurs when certain features of phonemes change, making the phonemes more similar to neighboring sounds. Assimilation can also include the addition or deletion of phonemes. Coarticulation, conversely, produces minor changes that may not be perceived by the listener. To understand the distinction between coarticulation and assimilation, consider the following. During the production of the word *sweet*, the *s* is produced with lip-rounding in anticipation of the normally rounded *w*, [s̫wit]. This modification is considered **coarticulation**, because one cannot perceive the alteration auditorily. However, when producing the phrase "and you go" /ænd ju go/, the /d/ and the /j/ sometimes change becoming the affricate /ʧ/, [ænʧu go]. This change can be detected auditorily; therefore, it is an **assimilation** process.

Additionally, the processes of **coarticulation** and **assimilation** can be classified as either **progressive** or **regressive** (Ladefoged, 2006). In **progressive assimilation,** a sound segment influences the sound following it. This type of sound change occurs in the word *horseshoe* /hɔrsʃu/. The /s/ at the end of *horse* is completely assimilated into the /ʃ/ in *shoe* and is pronounced [hɔrʃ:u] in connected speech. For **regressive assimilation**, a sound is changed due to the influence of a phoneme that follows it. Chapter 6's discussion of nasal speech sounds presented an example of **regressive assimilation.** Recall that when transcribing the nasal /n/ preceding a velar /k/, the velar position of the /k/ will influence the position of the nasal, causing it to become velar as well. For example, the word *pink* is not pronounced like the word *pin* with a *k* at the end /pɪnk/, but is articulated [pɪŋk]. This is an example of **regressive assimilation**.

The actual articulation of phonemes can also vary depending on where they appear within a word. For example, the voiceless stop /t/ will be produced with heavy aspiration if it releases a stressed syllable. Raise the back of your hand to your lips and say the word *top* /tɑp/. Did you feel the air hit the back of your hand as you released the /t/ in *top*? That air was the aspiration characteristic of a voiceless stop being released in the initial position of a stressed syllable. To indicate the heavily aspirated allophonic variation of the voiceless stop, the diacritic [ʰ] is added immediately following the stop [tʰɑp]. If, however, the voiceless stop is part of an *s*-cluster, the voiceless stop will be released but without heavy aspiration. Once again, place the back of your hand up to your mouth as you say *stop*. Notice this time that there is no heavy aspiration as you release the /t/. The narrow transcription indicating release without heavy aspiration is [st=ɑp]. Another allophonic variation as a result of phoneme placement is a voiceless stop at the end of a word. The final stop /t/ in the word *pot* will not normally be released in connected speech. Final stops are not typically released, irrespective of voicing. An example of the phonetic transcription indicating unreleased final stops is [pɑt̚]. Another example of allophonic variation resulting from phoneme position is alveolar stops following stressed vowels but preceding unstressed vowels. For example, in the word *pretty*, the intervocalic /t/ is produced as a flap [ɾ], i.e., it is made by the rapid raising and lowering of the tongue tip to the alveolar ridge. This type of production of both /t/ and its cognate /d/ is known as an alveolar flap, and the movements for its production is much more rapid than normally seen for /t/ or /d/. The narrow transcription of *pretty* produced with the flap would be [prɪɾi].

TRANSCRIBING ALLOPHONIC VARIATIONS

Now let's practice transcribing the allophonic variations using diacritics and special symbols to note the exact manner in which a phoneme is articulated. Recall that diacritic markings help in recording, as accurately as possible, the way that people speak and are vital in indicating allophonic variations that are a normal result of coarticulated speech. Narrow transcription can also be used to document disordered speech. Chapter 9 will focus on the use of diacritics and narrow transcription for recording disordered speech. The exercises presented in this chapter are intended to provide clarification on the dynamic nature of phonemes in connected speech. Keep in mind that SLPs primarily use diacritics and special notations only to document clinically relevant aspects of speech. Detailing all the phonetic elements of a client's speech would be an arduous and unnecessary task.

Narrow Transcription of the Stops

We will begin transcribing the allophonic variations of the stop phonemes discussed above. When the voiceless stops /p t k/ release stressed syllables, they are produced with heavy aspiration (puff of air). The diacritic indicating stop release with heavy aspiration is [^{h}].

Examples:

"kiss" →[k^{h}ɪs]

"team" →[t^{h}im]

"push"→[p^{h}ʊʃ]

Exercise 8.1 Transcribe the following words showing the heavy aspiration of voiceless stops:

1. key	[k^{h}i]	6. bane	[ben]
2. game	[gem]	7. touch	[t^{h}ʌtʃ]
3. Tom	[t^{h}am]	8. cash	[k^{h}æʃ]
4. pin	[p^{h}ɪn]	9. pear	[p^{h}ɛr]
5. car	[k^{h}ar]	10. dime	[daɪm]

Syllables releasing voiceless stops that are part of an *s-* cluster are released but without heavy aspiration. Voiceless stops are also released but without heavy aspiration when they appear in the onset position of an unstressed syllable. The diacritic marking indicating release of stops without heavy aspiration is [=].

Examples:

"skin" →[sk=ɪn]		"backup"→	[bæk=əp]
"steep" →[st=ip]		"flicker"→	[flɪk=ɚ]
"speech"→[sp=itʃ]		"twitter"→	[twɪt=ɚ]

Exercise 8.2 Transcribe the following words showing the release of voiceless stops without heavy aspiration:

1. sicker ______	6. whisker ______
2. spin ______	7. detail ______
3. speak ______	8. stain ______
4. star ______	9. scar ______
5. sky ______	10. checker ______

When voiced and voiceless stops appear in word-final position, they are often unreleased. Also in a sequence of two stops, the first one is typically not released. The diacritic marking used to indicate an unreleased stop is [˺].

Examples:

"sit" →[sɪt˺]	"mop bucket"→[mɑp˺bʌkɪt˺]
"mob →[mɑb˺]	"catnip"→[kæt˺nɪp˺]
"lad"→[læd˺]	"feet"→[fit˺]

Exercise 8.3 Transcribe the following words showing unreleased stops:

1. laptop ______	6. hope ______
2. skateboard ______	7. hog ______
3. sidecar ______	8. fig ______
4. mitt ______	9. sideboard ______
5. nope ______	10. leap ______

Exercise 8.4 Transcribe the following words showing the appropriate release and aspiration of all stops:

1. Razorback	[rezɚbæk˺]	6. date	[det˺]
2. pickpocket	[pʰɪk˺pʰak=ɛt˺]	7. stick	[st=ɪk˺]
3. steep	[st=ip˺]	8. custard	[kʰʌst=ɚd˺]
4. backpack	[bæk˺pʰæk˺]	9. Gamecock	[gemkʰak˺]
5. ductape	[dʌk˺tʰep˺]	10. stop	[st=ap˺]

Nasality

When nasals are produced in rapid speech, they will influence the vowels around them, causing the vowels to take on a nasal resonant quality. Most often, this occurs when the vowel sound is between two nasals or when the nasal is in word-final position. The velum will lower to produce or in anticipation of producing a nasal phoneme and remain lowered for articulation efficiency throughout the word. The diacritic to indicate nasality is [~], which is placed over the affected phoneme.

Examples:

"mom" → [mɑ̃m]

"moan"→ [mõn]

Exercise 8.5 Transcribe the following words, showing the influence of nasality on vowels:

1. Tom	[tɑ̃m]	6. pan	[pæ̃n]
2. tone	[tõn]	7. name	[nẽm]
3. tan	[tæ̃n]	8. Ming	[mɪ̃ŋ]
4. meme	[mɪ̃m]	9. can	[kæ̃n]
5. sing	[sɪ̃ŋ]	10. ma'am	[mæ̃m]

Dentalization

The alveolar consonants /t d s z n l/produced in rapid connected speech may shift in place of articulation and become dentalized, i.e., the tongue makes contact with the teeth rather than the alveolar ridge when occurring before either of the interdentals /θ ð/. The symbol to indicate dentalization is [̪], which is placed under the affected phoneme.

Examples:

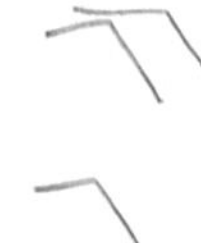

"eleventh " → [əˈlɛvən̪θ]

"unthinking" → [ən̪ˈθɪŋkɪŋ]

"width"→ [ˈwɪd̪θ]

Exercise 8.6 Transcribe the following words showing the dentalization of alveolar phonemes:

1. one that		6. on this	
2. synthetic		7. anthem	
3. enthuse		8. ninth	
4. menthol		9. Anthony	
5. panther		10. menthol	

Narrow Transcription of the Lateral Allophones

The production of the lateral /l/ is highly variable. The alveolar placement for the phoneme was introduced earlier in this text. The alveolar /l/ is known as the "clear" /l/ and is typically used in prevocalic productions. There is also the velarized /l/, which is made with an arching of the tongue in the velar region; this sound is most often used in postvocalic productions. The symbols for the clear /l/ and velar /l/ are [ʃ] and [L], respectively. SLPs should be aware of these differences in the production of the /l/ phoneme, particularly when developing lists of target words for treatment plans.

Examples:

"let" /lɛt/→[ʃɛt]	"milk" /mɪlk/→[mɪLk]
"lick" /lɪk/→[ʃɪk]	"curl" /kɝl/→[kɝL]
"lip" /lɪp/→[ʃɪp]	"dull" /dʌl/→[dʌL]

Exercise 8.7 Transcribe the following words showing the appropriate lateral allophone:

1. elk	[ɛLK]	6. loathe	[loð]
2. quell	[KWɛL]	7. Braille	[brɛL]
3. polka	[poLKə]	8. look	[lʊK]
4. oil	[ɔɪL]	9. led	[lɛd]
5. late	[let]	10. eel	[iL]

Devoicing of Liquids

When the liquid /l/ or /r/ appear in a consonant blend with either a voiceless stop or a voiceless fricative, the liquid will be devoiced; however, devoicing will not occur in a three-element blend, such as *–spl* or *–skr*. The diacritic marking to indicate devoicing is [̥] and is placed beneath the affected liquid.

Examples:

"plate" →[pl̥et]

"slip" →[sl̥ɪp]

"dream"→[dr̥im]

Exercise 8.8 Transcribe the following words showing the devoicing of liquids in voiceless stop and voiceless fricatives:

1. groom	[grum]	6. sleet	[sl̥it]
2. clue	[kl̥u]	7. plum	[pl̥ʌm]
3. floor	[fl̥ɔr]	8. pride	[pr̥aɪd]
4. slam	[sl̥æm]	9. stream	[strim]
5. blood	[blʌd]	10. tray	[tr̥e]

Alterations in Duration

Sometimes in connected speech, a word will end in the same phoneme that introduces the next word. When this occurs, the identical phoneme is not articulated twice; rather, the phoneme is just lengthened. The [:] diacritic is placed after the lengthened phoneme.

Examples:

"some more" →[sʌm:ɔr]

"good dog" →[gʊd:ɑg]

"fun night"→[fʌn:aɪt]

Exercise 8.9 Transcribe the following words showing lengthening of abutting phonemes:

1. fish shop	[fɪʃ:ɑp]	6. sweet talk	[swit:ɔlk]
2. hot tip	[hɑt:ɪp]	7. homemade	[hom:ed]
3. good day	[gʊd:e]	8. pick corn	[pɪk:ɔrn]
4. nice Sunday	[naɪs:ʌnde]	9. sit tall	[sɪt:ɔl]
5. blood donor	[blʌd:onɚ]	10. this soap	[ðɪs:op]

Transcribing Syllabic Consonants

In Chapter 1, the importance of syllabics was presented. Syllabics form the nucleus of a syllable, and thus every syllable must contain one (Shriberg & Kent, 1995). Typically, the nucleus of a syllable is a vowel; however, the liquid and nasal consonants can sometime serve as the nucleus of a syllable due to their vowel-like nature. The diacritic [ˌ] is placed under the liquid to identify the syllabic consonant and indicate that it is serving as the nucleus of a syllable. The syllabic /r/ is an exception to this, because the schwar /ɚ/ already demonstrates the vowel property of the /r/. The following shows how the vowel is subsumed in a syllabic consonant, causing it to function as both vowel and consonant.

/əm/ becomes /m̩/

/ən/ becomes /n̩/

/əl/ becomes /l̩/

/ər/ becomes /ɚ/

The /ŋ/ is not typically used as a syllabic, and the /m/ rarely is. Syllabic consonants will only appear in unstressed syllables; therefore, they will never occur in monosyllabic words.

Examples:

"rob 'em" →[rabm̩]

"molten" →[moltn̩]

"bottle"→[batL̩]

"sister"→[sɪstɚ]

You may have noted in the above examples that syllabic consonants often appear in homorganic conditions, that is, the consonant preceding the syllable consonant will have the same place of articulation (Kent, 1998). In the *rob 'em* [rabm̩] example, the *b* and *m* share the bilabial place of articulation; the *t* and *n* in *molten* [moltn̩] share the alveolar place of articulation, as do the *t* and *l* in *bottle* [batL̩]. This will not, however, hold true for the schwar /ɚ/.

Exercise 8.10 Transcribe the following words showing use of syllabic consonants:

1. middle	[mɪdL̩]	6. tattle	[tætL̩]
2. bitten	[bɪtn̩]	7. pillar	[pɪlɚ]
3. brittle	[brɪtL̩]	8. mitten	[mɪtn̩]
4. brother	[brʌðɚ]	9. kettle	[kɛtL̩]
5. panel	[pænL̩]	10. dimple	[dɪmpL̩]

Glottal Stops

The glottal stop [ʔ] is a stop phoneme that is made at the glottis by rapidly narrowing and briefly closing the vocal folds. It is most often heard in American English as an allophone of /t/ appearing before a syllabic consonant [n̩]. Our friends "across the pond" might also use this dialectical variation when /t/ occurs before the syllabic /l/, as in bottle [baʔL̩].

Examples:

"kitten" →[kɪʔn̩]

"patent" →[pæʔn̩t]

"bitten"→[bɪʔn̩]

Exercise 8.11 Transcribe the following words showing use of glottal stops before syllabic consonants:

1. button	[bʌʔn̩]	6. lighten	[laɪʔn̩]
2. mitten	[mɪʔn̩]	7. fittin'	[fɪʔn̩]
3. Latin	[læʔn̩]	8. mutton	[mʌʔn̩]
4. fatten	[fæʔn̩]	9. satin	[sæʔn̩]
5. batten	[bæʔn̩]	10. written	[rɪʔn̩]

Partial Voicing of Intervocalic /t/

When the /t/ occurs between two vowels (intervocalic), it is oftentimes partially voiced due to the influence of the voiced vowels surrounding it. Sometimes the assimilation is so great that the /t/ will be completely voiced and become a /d/. When complete voicing occurs, the /d/ phoneme can be transcribed, but when the /t/ phoneme is produced with partial voicing, the diacritic indicating partial voicing [̬] is used.

Examples:

"gritted" →[grɪt̬ɛd]

"limited" →[lɪmt̬ɛd]

"bloated"→[blot̬əd]

Exercise 8.12 Transcribe the following words showing partial voicing of the intervocalic /t/:

1. metal	[mɛt̬l̩]	6. litter	[lɪt̬ɚ]
2. latter	[læt̬ɚ]	7. pretty	[prɪt̬i]
3. bitter	[bɪt̬ɚ]	8. letter	[lɛt̬ɚ]
4. butter	[bʌt̬ɚ]	9. later	[let̬ɚ]
5. atom	[æt̬m̩]	10. pattern	[pæt̬ɚn]

Alternately, the intervocalic /t/, and the /d/, can be produced with the alveolar flap, which is a variant produced by the rapid raising and lowering of the tongue to the alveolar ridge. The diacritic indicating the flap is [ɾ]. Don't be concerned if you are unable to differentiate among the [t̬], [d], and [ɾ] productions. The distinction is hard to determine, because acoustically, the sounds are very similar.

PHONOTACTICS

This text has presented the contrastive phonemes of English and the symbols used to transcribe them. This chapter has dealt with the variations of these phonemes (allophones) due to the influence of neighboring speech sounds and the position in a word in which phonemes appear. However, not all phoneme segments can occur as the onsets and codas of syllables. The rules for the permissible combination of sound segments to form syllables are known as phonotactics (O'Grady, Archibald, Aronoff and Rees-Miller, 2001). Try pronouncing the following lists:

List A	**List B**
Trasp	Mgla
Splemt	Vprog
Plunt	Zhizn

Was it easier to pronounce List A than List B? List A is easier, because, although the content of List A does not contain real words, the sound combinations used to construct the non-words conform to the phonotactic rules of English, making it possible to pronounce them. List B contains actual Russian words that don't conform to English phonotactic rules, making them difficult for English speakers to pronounce. According to O'Grady, Archibald, Aronoff, and Rees-Miller (2001) "Each language has its own set of restrictions on the phonological shapes of its syllable constituents" (p. 83). Every language has a finite set of phonemes and a method for how these phonemes can be arranged to form words.

Pena-Brooks and Hegde (2000) outlined examples of phonotactic rules for English. There are rules governing where individual phonemes may appear, rules dictating which phonemes may be combined, and rules describing the number of consonants that can be combined at the beginning and ending of words.

Let's take a look at these phonotactic constraints with some examples of how they apply to our language. The first rule outlines where sounds can occur. In English, talkers are permitted to begin words with glides as in *wait /wet/* and *yea /ye/*; speakers, however, are not allowed to end words with a glide. Note the word *paw* is orthographically written with the grapheme *w* at the end; however, the *w* is silent, because the word is pronounced */pɔ/*, not */pɔw/*. Try to pronounce it with the glide at the end, and you will discover how awkward it is.

Another rule dictates how phonemes may be combined. It is permissible to combine */tr- /*, */sp-/*, and */bl-/* at the beginning of words, as in *tray /tre/*, *slay /sle/*, and *blame /blem/*. It is not permissible for these combinations to be used at the ends of words. However, English speakers may combine the consonants */-sp/*, */-rm/*, and */-st/* at the end of words as in *clasp /klæsp/*, *farm/farm/*, and *pest /pɛst/*.

The final phonotactic rule outlines the number of consonants that may be combined to form clusters. English speakers may combine two and three consonants at the beginning of words, such as *spay /spe/*, and *screw /skru/* and up to four consonants may be combined at the end of words, although this is rare. The word *glimpsed /glɪmpst/* is an example of four consonants combined to form a cluster in the final position.

MORPHOPHONEMICS

In orthography, consistent spellings of plural and past tense suffixes are used even though the phonemes may vary. Sound alterations occur when free and bound morphemes combine, and there are rules detailing their combination known as morphophonemics (Peña-Brooks and Hegde, 2000). The following are examples of morphophonemic rules for making nouns plural and for showing verb tense in English.

When a free morpheme (noun) is made plural, its final sound will determine the attached morpheme. If the free morpheme ends in a voiceless sound, then the attached morpheme will also be voiceless, i.e., */s/.* For example, *pot* ends in the voiceless */t/,* therefore, the attached morpheme will be the voiceless */s/* as in *pot + s= pots /pats/.* If the free morpheme ends in a voiced sound, then the attached morpheme will also be voiced, i.e., */z/* will be produced as in *dog + s= dogs /dagz/.* If the free morpheme being made plural already ends in an *s* or *z* or other *sibilant*, the attached morpheme */ɛz/* or */ɪz/* will be used as in *bus+es= busses /bʌsɛz/* or */bʌsɪz/.* Note that this rule applies to any free morpheme ending in a sibilant, for example, *witch+es = witches /wɪʧɛz/* or */wɪʧɪz/.*

Exercise 8.13 Make the following nouns plural:

1. hog [hagz]	11. wreath [riθs]
2. girl [gɝlz]	12. herb [ɝbz]
3. shoe [ʃuz]	13. letter [lɛtɚz]
4. sloth [slaθs]	14. judge [dʒʌdʒɪz]
5. birthmark [bɝθmarks]	15. pattern [pætɚnz]
6. bush [bʊʃɪz]	16. plate [plets]
7. chair [tʃɛrz]	17. pillow [pɪloz]
8. couch [koʊtʃɪz]	18. one [wʌnz]
9. rug [rʌgz]	19. tube [tubz]
10. boat [bots]	20. clock [klaks]

There are also guidelines for making verbs past tense, and these rules also rely on the voicing elements of the morphemes to be combined. For example, if a verb ends in a voiceless sound, the attached morpheme will also be voiceless.

- *Pop + ed = popped,* which is pronounced */papt/.*

If a verb ends in a voiced sound, the attached morpheme will also be voiced.

- *Play + ed = played,* which is pronounced */pled/.*

If a verb ends in a */t/* or */d/,* the attached morpheme will be */ɛd/* or */ɪd/,* depending on pronunciation.

- *Vote + ed= voted,* which is pronounced */votɛd/* or */votɪd/.*

Exercise 8.14 Make the following verbs past tense:

1. smooth [smuðd]
2. hop [hapt]
3. buzz [bʌzd]
4. ask [æskt]
5. follow [falod]
6. alert [əlɛ˞tɪd]
7. blush [blʌʃt]
8. chew [tʃud]
9. brake [brekt]
10. stop [stapt]
11. include [ɪnkludɛd]
12. need [nidɛd]
13. work [wɝkt]
14. seem [simd]
15. camp [kæmpt]
16. cheat [tʃitɛd]
17. beg [bɛgd]
18. arrest [ərɛstɛd]

CONCLUSION

Although it is not necessary to transcribe allophonic variations that occur as a part of normal coarticulation of connected speech, it is important for the speech-language pathologist to understand these processes and the dynamic nature of speech production in order to effectively manage speech sound disorders. Additionally, the phonotactic rules for how sound segments combine, as well as the morphophonemic alterations that occur when free and bound morphemes combine, provide a foundation for understanding the sound system of our language and the rules for modifying it.

CHAPTER

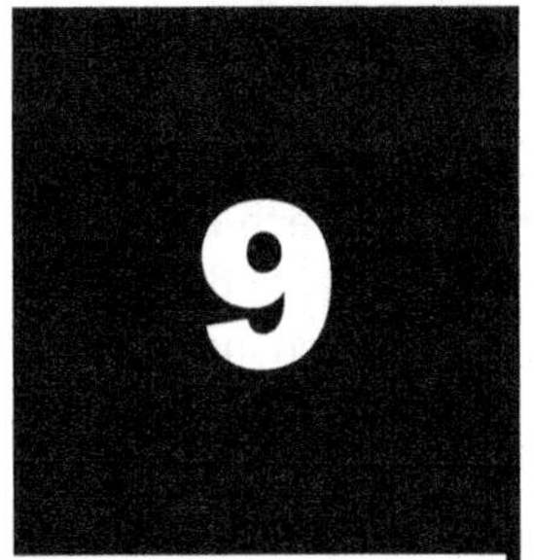

Chapter 8 focused on the normal changes to phonemes that result from coarticulation and assimilation. Chapters 9 and 10 will delve into transcribing and analyzing disordered speech. These chapters will present the opportunity for you to put into practice the skills presented thus far in this text. Although there is no clear consensus among researchers regarding the categorization of speech sound disorders, in terms of describing sound errors, this text will focus on three classifications: articulation (also known as phonetic), phonological (also known as phonemic), and childhood apraxia of speech (CAS).

TRANSCRIBING DISORDERED SPEECH

Articulation (phonetic) disorders refer to errors in the production of phonemes that result from problems in speech motor control. Children exhibiting articulation difficulties will usually have mild-to-moderate impairment characterized by problems producing certain phonemes (Van Riper & Smith, 1979). For example, a child with articulation disorder may have trouble coordinating the tongue for the correct production of the /r/ phoneme. These errors are typically consistent.

Phonological (phonemic) disorders have a cognitive-linguistic origin in which children have difficulty developing and using the language rules that underlie speech. This designation focuses on the child's use of phoneme contrasts, constraints, and phonological patterns. Phonological disorders will be the focus of Chapter 10.

CAS refers to sound errors that involve motor planning and/or programming issues. According to the American Speech-Language-Hearing Association's (ASHA's) 2007 position statement, CAS is a neurological speech sound disorder presenting in childhood. Although this text will not address CAS specifically, the notations and transcription rules offered in this chapter and the next will also be useful when documenting the speech of a child with suspected CAS.

TRANSCRIBING PHONETIC DISORDERS

Although phonetic (narrow) transcription can be used to indicate allophonic variations, it is unnecessary and too time consuming to include all the phonetic details of a client's speech, particularly those details that correspond to normal coarticulation and assimilatory processes. However, for the speech-language pathologist (SLP), phonetic transcription is a powerful tool to document the clinically relevant aspects of disordered speech. It is usually recommended that square brackets be used in phonetic transcription when indicating error productions.

There are a number of different types of speech sound errors and ways to notate the errors: substitutions, omissions, distortions, and additions (Van Riper & Erickson, 1979). The following is a description of speech sound error types:

SUBSTITUTION

Substitutions are the most common type of speech errors and occur when one sound is substituted for another sound. An example would be [tæt] for [kæt]; the /t/ is substituted for the /k/. There are different ways to denote a sound substitution:

x→y means "x becomes y."

y/x means "y for x."

x→y/z means "x becomes y in the environment of z." This symbolization describes how a phonetic or word context influences speech production.

The above notations provide a convenient mechanism to describe speech sound changes.

OMISSION

An omission occurs when a speech sound in a target word is not produced. An example would be [bʌ] for [bʌs].

DISTORTION

An allophone is produced for the intended phoneme. An example would be the dentalized or frontal /s/, in the word [s̪ʌn].

ADDITION

The insertion of an extra sound in a word. An example would be the /ə/ in the word [bəlæk].

NARROW TRANSCRIPTION OF PHONETIC DISORDERS

Nasal Symbols

The following are symbols used to signal changes in the nasality of speech (Bauman-Wängler, 2012).

Hypernasality

Hypernasality describes deviant nasal resonance affecting vowels and vocalic consonants (oral resonant consonants). Hypernasality results from coupling of the oral and nasal cavities due to problems with velopharyngeal closure. The diacritic to indicate hypernasality is the tilde [~] placed above the affected phoneme.

Examples:

"water" /watɚ/→[w̃ãtɚ̃]

"yuck" /jʌk/→[j̃ʌ̃k]

" yep" /jɛp/→[j̃ɛ̃p]

Exercise 9.1 Transcribe the following words to show the presence of hypernasality:

1. wet	[w̃ɛ̃t]	6. feud	[f̃j̃ũd]
2. your	[j̃ɔ̃r̃]	7. quit	[kw̃ɪ̃t]
3. weed	[w̃ĩd]	8. we	[w̃ĩ]
4. way	[w̃ẽ]	9. wake	[w̃ẽk]
5. stress	[s̃tr̃ɛ̃s̃]	10. yard	[j̃ãr̃d]

Nasal Emission

Nasal emission is deviant airflow and emission through the nose on the production of pressure consonants, i.e., stops, fricatives, and affricates. Like hypernasality, nasal emission results from inappropriate coupling of the oral and nasal cavities. The diacritic to indicate nasal emission is the [⃰] placed above the affected phoneme.

Examples:

"pop" /pap/→[p⃰ap⃰]

"soap" /sop/→[s⃰op⃰]

"chip" /ʧɪp/→[ʧ⃰ɪp⃰]

Exercise 9.2 Transcribe the following words to show the presence of nasal emission:

1. chick	[t͡ʃ͋ɪk͋]	6. juice	[d͡ʒ͋us͋]
2. pup	[p͋ʌp͋]	7. pot	[p͋ɑt͋]
3. shoe	[ʃ͋u]	8. ship	[ʃ͋ɪp͋]
4. shut	[ʃ͋ʌt͋]	9. zoo	[ʒ͋u]
5. big	[b͋ɪg͋]	10. peach	[p͋it͡ʃ͋]

Hyponasality (Denasality)

Hyponasality describes the reduction of nasal quality. Only nasal consonants can be denasalized. Hyponasality is most often associated with the way people sound when they have a cold (Small, 2005). For example, the phrase "My mom is Nona" may sound like "By bob is Doda." The diacritic to indicate hyponasality is the tilde with a slash through it [͊] placed above the affected phoneme.

Examples:

"mop" /mɑp/→[m͊ɑp]

"tan" /tæn/→[tæn͊]

"pink" / pɪŋk /→[pɪŋ͊k]

Exercise 9.3 Transcribe the following words to show the presence of hyponasality:

1. none	[n͊ʌn͊]	6. game	[gem͊]
2. mean	[m͊in͊]	7. matt	[m͊æt]
3. name	[n͊em͊]	8. fun	[fʌn͊]
4. sing	[sɪŋ͊]	9. mutts	[m͊ʌts]
5. birthmark	[bɝθm͊ark]	10. pattern	[pætən͊]

Tongue Symbols

The following are tongue symbols used to signal deviations from typical tongue placement for consonant speech sounds.

Frontal Lisp

For the /s/ and /z/ phonemes, the typical alveolar tongue placement is shifted slightly forward toward the upper incisors, causing the sounds to become dentalized. The diacritic marking this placement shift is [̪] placed under the affected phoneme.

Examples:

"sun" /sʌn/→[s̪ʌn]

"zoo" /zu/→[z̪u]

"plus" / plʌs /→[plʌs̪]

Exercise 9.4 Transcribe the following words to show the presence of a frontal lisp:

1. zip	[z̪ɪp]	6. buzz	[bʌz̪]
2. cousin	[kʌz̪ɛn]	7. pencil	[pɛns̪əL]
3. blossom	[blas̪əm]	8. pose	[poz̪]
4. soul	[s̪oL]	9. sank	[s̪æŋk]
5. south	[s̪aʊθ]	10. city	[s̪ɪti]

Lateral Lisp

For this error production, the tongue is generally in position to produce the clear /l/, but the airflow is released with friction laterally into the checks. The symbols for /s/ and /z/ are [ʪ] and [ʫ], respectively.

Examples:

"sun" /sʌn/→[ʪʌn]

"zoo" /zu/→[ʫu]

"plus" / plʌs /→[plʌʪ]

Exercise 9.5 Transcribe the following words to show the presence of a lateral lisp:

1. seven	[ɬɛvən]	6. stanza	[ɬtænɮə]
2. Samantha	[ɬəmænθə]	7. silly	[ɬɪli]
3. fancy	[fænɬi]	8. graze	[greɮ]
4. satire	[ɬætaɪr]	9. czar	[ɮar]
5. hose	[hoɮ]	10. cedar	[ɬidɚ]

Palatal

This notation indicates the presence of an /s/ or /z/ phoneme that is produced with a slight place shift to a slightly more posterior tongue position that approaches that of the /ʃ/. The symbol for a palatial /s/ or /z/ is [sʲ] or [zʲ], respectively.

Examples:

"sun" /sʌn/→[sʲʌn]

"zoo" /zu/→[zʲu]

"plus" / plʌs /→[plʌsʲ]

Exercise 9.6 Transcribe the following words to show the presence of a palatal /s/:

1. zipper	[zʲɪpɚ]	6. lazy	[lezʲi]
2. sink	[sʲɪŋk]	7. scissors	[sʲɪzʲɚzʲ]
3. Sue	[sʲu]	8. zeal	[zʲil]
4. soap	[sʲop]	9. Xanadu	[zʲænədu]
5. zone	[zʲon]	10. moose	[musʲ]

CONCLUSION

Phonetic (narrow) transcription is a powerful tool for the SLP. It offers an efficient and convenient mechanism to record the clinically relevant aspects of a client's speech.

CHAPTER

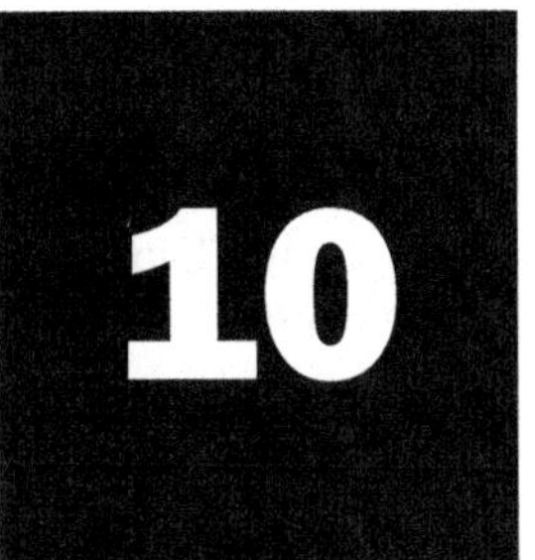

Research in the area of sound acquisition has revealed that children simplify adult forms of words in consistent ways to make speech easier to produce while their motoric systems and language rule systems develop. Phonological error patterns have been identified to describe the changes that children make. These alterations affect classes of sounds and/or the syllabic structure of words. There are many error patterns described in the literature. Some are a normal or "natural" part of development, while others are not. In their 1980 review, Shriberg and Kwiatkowski identified more than 40 natural processes. Ingram (1981) arranged error patterns into three broad categories. The first category is syllable structure patterns in which children alter the syllabic structure of words, such as producing a singleton consonant rather than a consonant cluster, for example *[pun]* instead of */spun/.* Sound substitution patterns describe the replacement of one class of phonemes for another. Usually earlier developing classes are exchanged for later developing ones, such as substituting a stop for a fricative, for example *[tup]* for */sup/.* Assimilation patterns refer to children's attempt to make the target word easier to produce by making all the consonants in a word similar, for example *[lɛlo]* for */jɛlo/.* This is also known as consonant harmony. The concept of these simplification patterns was derived from research on children's word use during the first few years of life. Although there are differences in the terminology used to describe error patterns by various authors, this chapter presents patterns most typically seen in the literature and follows those presented by Stoel-Gammon and Dunn (1985).

TRANSCRIBING PHONEMIC DISORDERS

Determining if a child is using phonological error patterns is an important part of the assessment and analysis of a child's speech. Speech-language pathologists (SLPs) analyze speech by reviewing errors to determine if commonalities exist among them that form patterns. The exercises presented in this chapter will put to use not only your knowledge of manner, place, and voice, but also your understanding of distinctive features. This chapter is an exciting one to explore, because you will have the opportunity to apply the knowledge and skills learned in this text to the actual analysis of speech disorders.

Phonological Simplification Patterns

Syllable Structure Simplification Patterns

Children will change the syllable structure of a word to make it easier to say. Children will either alter the number of syllables of a multisyllabic word or change the syllable shape of the word.

Weak Syllable Deletion

This pattern only occurs with multisyllabic words. Children will typically omit the unstressed or "weak" syllable of a word. Usually, the unstressed syllable will be at the beginning of a word or in the middle of the word.

Examples:

"computer" /kəmpjutɚ/→[pjutɚ]

"telephone" /tɛləfon/→[tɛfon]

"banana" /bənænə/→[nænə]

Exercise 10.1 Transcribe the following words showing weak syllable deletion.

1. tomato	[medo]	6. surprise	[paɪz]
2. spaghetti	[gɛti]	7. refrigerator	[frɪdʒretɚ]
3. spider web	[spaɪwɛb]	8. pajamas	[dʒaməz]
4. dinosaur	[daɪsɔr]	9. helicopter	[hɛlkaptɚ]
5. vitamin	[vaɪmɪn]	10. watermelon	[wamɛlən]

Final Consonant Deletion

This is a very common error pattern in which children omit a final singleton consonant, resulting in a target word ending in an open syllable.

Examples:

"boot" /but/→[bu]

"cup" /kʌp/→[kʌ]

"push" /pʊʃ/→[pʊ]

Initial Consonant Deletion

This pattern is not as common as Final Consonant Deletion, and it is not considered a natural pattern or one that is seen in normal development. As the name implies, the initial singleton consonant is deleted.

Examples:

"fish" /fɪʃ/→[ɪʃ]

"cup" /kʌp/→[ʌp]

"top" /tɑp/→[ɑp]

Exercise 10.2 Transcribe the following words showing the effect of final consonant deletion (FCD) or initial consonant deletion (ICD). If one of these error patterns is not possible, write NP:

Target:	**FCD**	**ICD**
1. shoe	NP	[u]
2. Jeff	[dʒɛ]	[ɛf]
3. nope	[no]	[op]
4. though	NP	[o]
5. eat	[i]	NP
6. mash	[mæ]	[æʃ]
7. say	NP	[e]
8. kite	[kaɪ]	[aɪt]
9. cop	[kɑ]	[ɑp]
10. juice	[dʒu]	[us]

Epenthesis

Typically, epenthesis is the insertion of a vowel, usually the schwa, between a consonant cluster, resulting in an extra syllable in the word. The addition of the schwa between a consonant cluster simplifies the production of the cluster. Epenthesis can occur when any extra phoneme, be it consonant or vowel, is inserted in a word, but it most typically occurs when the schwa is inserted.

Examples:

"blue" /blu/→[bəlu]

"plate" /plet/→[pəlet]

"spy" /spaɪ/→[səpaɪ]

Exercise 10.3 Transcribe the following words showing epenthesis:

1. spoon	[səpun]	6. please	[pəliz]
2. spot	[səpat]	7. crown	[kəraʊn]
3. black	[bəlæk]	8. stop	[sətap]
4. tree	[təri]	9. trapper	[təræpɚ]
5. grape	[gərep]	10. play	[pəle]

Reduplication

This pattern occurs when a syllable is completely or partially repeated. Sometimes this pattern is referred to as "doubling."

Examples:

"bottle" /bɑtəl/→[bɑbɑ]

"water" /wɑtɚ/→[wɑwɑ]

"basket" /bæskət/→[bæbæ]

Exercise 10.4 Transcribe the following words showing reduplication:

1. cookie	[kʊkʊ]	6. blanket	[blæŋkblæŋk]
2. mitten	[mɪmɪ]	7. television	[tɛltɛl]
3. supper	[sʌpsʌp]	8. zipper	[zɪpzɪp]
4. napkin	[næpnæp]	9. butter	[bʌbʌ]
5. pillow	[pɪlpɪl]	10. middle	[mɪmɪ]

Diminutization

Diminutization occurs when [i] is inserted at the end of a word, resulting in an extra syllable in a word.

Examples:

"boot" /but/→[buti]

"dog" /dɑg/→[dɑgi]

"horse" /hɔrs/→[hɔrsi]

Exercise 10.5 Transcribe the following words showing diminutization.

1. hog	[hagi]	6. soap	[sopi]
2. cup	[kʌpi]	7. comb	[komi]
3. doll	[dɔli]	8. bath	[bæθi]
4. coat	[koti]	9. clown	[klaʊni]
5. lamp	[læmpi]	10. juice	[dʒusi]

Cluster Reduction or Deletion

These patterns occur when children attempt to simplify a consonant cluster by omitting a part of it or the whole cluster. Typically, the most difficult to produce consonant will be the one omitted.

Examples:

"blu" /blu/→[bu] *(cluster reduction)*

"stripe" /straɪp/→[taɪp] *(cluster reduction)*

"post" /post/→[po] *(cluster deletion)*

Exercise 10.6 Transcribe the following words showing cluster reduction or deletion. If cluster reduction or deletion is not possible for the word, write NP:

1. snow	[no]	6. tack	NP
2. skate	[ket]	7. jump	[dʒʌ]
3. star	[tar]	8. glue	[gu]
4. black	[bæk]	9. wish	NP
5. path	NP	10. beast	[bit]

Substitution Simplification Patterns

The most common type of simplification patterns is sound substitution patterns. These occur when one sound is substituted for another sound, independent of phonetic context, i.e., the sound change is not due to assimilation. In order to be considered a substitution pattern, there must be a systematic sound change that affects classes of sounds or sound sequences.

Stopping

Stopping occurs when a stop replaces a fricative or an affricate. Typically, the substituted stop will have the same manner of articulation and voicing as the target sound that it replaces.

Examples:

"sew" /so/→[to]

"fat" /fæt/→[pæt]

"push" /puʃ/→[pʊt]

Exercise 10.7 Transcribe the following words showing stopping:

1. shut	[tʌt]	6. shoe	[tu]
2. juice	[du]	7. sun	[tʌn]
3. thirsty	[dɝti]	8. ship	[tɪp]
4. soup	[tup]	9. zipper	[dɪpɚ]
5. fish	[pɪt]	10. vase	[bet]

Stridency Deletion

This simplification pattern includes the substitution of a strident phoneme with a non-strident sound or the deletion of a strident sound.

Examples:

"soup" /sup/→[θup]

"soup" /sup/→[tup]

"soup" /sup/→[up]

Exercise 10.8 Transcribe the following words showing stridency deletion:

1. hush	[hʌt]	6. cash	[kæt]
2. zoo	[du]	7. Sue	[tu]
3. thief	[θi]	8. finger	[tɪŋɚ]
4. sugar	[ʌgɚ]	9. vet	[bɛt]
5. pencil	[pɛntvl]	10. gross	[gro]

Fronting

This pattern involves place of articulation. Palatal and velar sounds /ʧ ʤ ʃ ʒ k g ŋ/ are replaced with sounds with a more anterior placement, most commonly the stops /t/ and /d/.

Examples:

"shoe" /ʃu/→[tu]

"go" /go/→[to]

"sing" /sɪŋ/→[sɪn]

Exercise 10.9 Transcribe the following words showing fronting:

1. show	[to]	6. juice	[dus]
2. game	[dem]	7. hog	[had]
3. goat	[dot]	8. kitten	[tɪʔ]
4. car	[tar]	9. cake	[tet]
5. cape	[tep]	10. girl	[dɝl]

Depalatalization

For this pattern, a palatal obstruent sound is replaced by a more anterior nonpalatal obstruent sound.

Examples:

"shoe" /ʃu/→[tu]

"beige" /beʒ/→[bed]

"chick" /ʧɪk/→[sɪk]

Exercise 10.10 Transcribe the following words showing depalatalization.

1. wash	[wat]	6. church	[tɝt]
2. shut	[tʌt]	7. judge	[dʌd]
3. juice	[dus]	8. beige	[bed]
4. push	[pʌt]	9. shoot	[ʃut]
5. ship	[tɪp]	10. wish	[wɪʃ]

Alveolarization

This pattern describes a minor place shift from the lips or teeth to the alveolar ridge. The sound substitution will only involve obstruents.

Examples:

"buy" /baɪ/→[daɪ]

"think" /θɪŋk/→[tɪŋk]

"fat" /fæt/→[tæt]

Exercise 10.11 Transcribe the following words showing alveolarization:

1. pear	[tɛr]	6. thought	[tat]
2. bear	[dɛr]	7. thin	[tɪn]
3. thing	[tɪŋ]	8. pig	[tɪg]
4. vase	[des]	9. bat	[dæt]
5. thirsty	[tɝsti]	10. fat	[tæt]

Labialization

This pattern also describes a minor place shift from the alveolar ridge or teeth to the lips. Similar to alveolarization, labialization only involves obstruents.

Examples:

"dog" /dɑg/→[bɑg]

"think" /θɪŋk/→[pɪŋk]

"sun" /sʌn/→[pʌn]

Exercise 10.12 Transcribe the following words showing labialization:

1. tap	[pæp]	6. thick	[pɪk]
2. tore	[pɔr]	7. thigh	[paɪ]
3. door	[bɔr]	8. tan	[pæn]
4. dear	[bir]	9. soap	[pop]
5. thank	[peŋk]	10. sick	[pɪk]

Gliding

This pattern involves the replacement of liquids with glides and is a very common error pattern among young children.

Examples:

"rock" /rɑk/→[wɑk]

"lip" /lɪp/→[wɪp]

"lick" /lɪk/→[jɪk]

Exercise 10.13 Transcribe the following words showing gliding:

1. lake	[jek]	6. rope	[wop]
2. lady	[wedi]	7. carrot	[kɛwət]
3. rabbit	[wæbɪt]	8. leg	[jɛg]
4. like	[jaɪk]	9. yellow	[jɛjo]
5. rat	[wæt]	10. leap	[wip]

Vowelization

Also called vocalization, this pattern occurs when syllabic liquids or nasals, rhotic diphthongs, rhotic central vowels, or velar [L] sounds are replaced with vowels. The vowels most commonly substituted are [ə], [o], and [ʊ].

Examples:

"sister" /sɪstɚ/→[sɪstə]

"bottle" /bɑtəl/→[bɑto]

"pear" /pɛr/→[pɛə]

Exercise 10.14 Transcribe the following words showing vowelization:

1. car	[kɑə]	4. little	[lɪto]
2. tiger	[taɪgə]	5. burn	[bʌn]
3. model	[mɑdo]	6. sister	[sɪstə]

7. mother	[mʌbə]	9. table	[tebo]
8. star	[sta]	10. bigger	[bɪgə]

Assimilation Simplification Patterns

Also called consonant harmony, assimilation simplification patterns describe a sound becoming more like a neighboring sound, i.e., the sound change is due to the influence of phonetic context (MacKay, 1987).

Labial Assimilation

This assimilation occurs when a sound changes to a labial due to the influence of another labial in the word. It can be complete or partial and progressive or regressive.

Examples:

"boot" /but/→[bup] (partial, progressive)

"hop" /hɑp/→[pɑp] (complete, regressive)

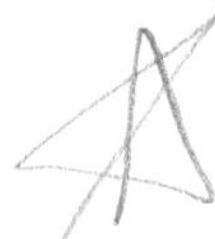

"top" /tɑp/→[pɑp] (partial, regressive)

Exercise 10.15 Transcribe the following words showing labial assimilation:

1. bat	[bæp]	6. hop	[pap]
2. fat	[fæp]	7. home	[pom]
3. boot	[bup]	8. book	[bʊm]
4. mitt	[mɪp]	9. make	[mep]
5. moat	[mop]	10. pan	[pæp]

Alveolar Assimilation

This assimilation occurs when a sound changes to a alveolar due to the influence of another alveolar in the word.

Examples:

"cat" /kæt/→[tæt] (complete regressive)

"top" /tɑp/→[tɑt] (complete progressive)

"deck" /dɛk/→[dɛt] (partial progressive)

Exercise 10.16 Transcribe the following words showing alveolar assimilation:

1. got	[dɑt]	6. dig	[dɪd]
2. tip	[tɪd]	7. hit	[dɪt]
3. Maddie	[dædi]	8. pot	[tɑt]
4. fat	[tæt]	9. top	[tɑt]
5. nope	[not]	10. cheat	[tit]

Velar Assimilation

This assimilation occurs when a sound changes to a velar due to the influence of another velar in the word.

Examples:

"cat" /kæt/→[kæg] (partial progressive)

"take" /tek/→[kek] (complete regressive)

"sing" /sɪŋ/→[kɪŋ] (partial regressive)

Exercise 10.17 Transcribe the following words showing velar assimilation:

1. keep	[kik]	6. park	[kark]
2. gate	[gek]	7. hog	[kag]
3. goat	[gok]	8. fig	[gɪg]
4. kiss	[kɪk]	9. fork	[kɔrk]
5. pick	[gɪk]	10. Kim	[kɪg]

Nasal Assimilation

This assimilation occurs when a sound changes to a nasal due to the influence of another nasal in the word.

Examples:

"pan" /pæn/→[næn] (complete regressive)

"mat" /mæt/→[mæn] (partial progressive)

"sing" /sɪŋ/→[nɪŋ] (partial regressive)

Exercise 10.18 Transcribe the following words showing nasal assimilation:

1. map	[mæn]	6. phone	[mon]
2. pink	[nɪŋk]	7. fame	[mem]
3. Pam	[mæm]	8. mate	[mæn]
4. tone	[non]	9. note	[non]
5. nope	[non]	10. more	[mon]

Prevocalic Voicing

This pattern results when voiceless obstruents preceding vowels become voiced.

Examples:

"cap" /kæp/→[gap]

"sun" /sʌn/→[zʌn]

"chip" /ʧɪp/→[ʤɪp]

Exercise 10.19 Transcribe the following words showing prevocalic voicing:

1. take	[dek]	6. tiger	[dɪgɚ]
2. pan	[bæn]	7. cow	[gaʊ]
3. soap	[zop]	8. pain	[ben]
4. ship	[dʒɪp]	9. chair	[dʒɝ]
5. sit	[zɪt]	10. cake	[gek]

Postvocalic Devoicing

This pattern occurs when a voiced obstruent in the final position of a word becomes voiceless.

Examples:

"paid" /ped/→[pet]

"dog" /dɑg/→[dɑk]

"five" /faɪv/→[faɪf]

Exercise 10.20 Transcribe the following words showing postvocalic devoicing:

1. rag	[ræk]	6. Hogue	[hok]
2. skid	[skɪt]	7. hog	[hɑk]
3. side	[saɪt]	8. maze	[mes]
4. pad	[pæt]	9. jab	[dʒæp]
5. knob	[nɑp]	10. made	[met]

CONCLUSION

Phonological analysis of children's speech is a crucial aspect of speech-language pathology. The exercises presented in this chapter were designed to give you a sample of the work you will be engaged in once you are a practicing professional. The activities were also designed to highlight the importance of the information that has been presented in this text.

REFERENCES

Bauman-Wängler, J. A. (2012). *Articulatory and phonological impairments: A clinical focus.* Boston, MA: Pearson.

Bernhardt, B., & Stoel-Gammon, C. (1994). Nonlinear phonology: Introduction and clinical application. *Journal of Speech and Hearing Research, 37*(1), 123–143.

Chomsky, N., & M. Halle (1968). *The sound pattern of English.* New York, NY: Harper & Row.

Dirckx, J.H. (1997). Medical Meanings: A Glossary of Word Origins. *JAMA: The Journal of the American Medical Association*, 278(8), 688.

Dodd, B., & Gillon, G. (2001). Exploring the relationship between phonological awareness, speech impairment and literacy. *Advances in Speech Language Pathology, 3*(2), 139–147.

Edwards, H. T. (2003). *Applied phonetics: The sounds of American English.* New York, NY: Delmar Learning.

Edwards, M. L., & Shriberg, L. D. (1983). Issues in phonological assessment. *Seminars in Speech and Language,* 4, 351–374.

Eimas, P. D., Siqueland, E. R., Jusczyk, P., & Vigorito, J. (1971). Speech Perception in Infants. *Science*, 171(3968), 303-306.

Fry, D. B. (1955). Duration and intensity as physical correlates of linguistic stress. *Journal Acoustical Society of America*, 27, 765–768.

Gerken, L., & McGregor, K.K. (1998). An overview of prosody and its role in normal and disordered child language. *American Journal of Speech-Language Pathology,* 7, 38–48.

Grunwell, P. (1987). *Clinical phonology* (2nd ed.). London, UK: Croom Helm.

Hanna, P. R., Hanna, J. S., Hodges, R. E., & Rudorf, E. H. (1966). *Phoneme-grapheme correspondences as cues to spelling improvement.* Washington, DC: U.S. Department of Health, Education, and Welfare.

Hodson, B. (1997). Disordered phonologies: What have we learned about assessment and treatment? In B. Hodson & M. Edwards (Eds.), *Perspectives in applied phonology* (pp. 197–224). New York, NY: Aspen Publishers.

Hodson, B., & Strattman, K. (2004). Phonological awareness intervention for children with expressive phonological impairments. In R. Kent (Ed.). *The MIT encyclopedia of communication disorders* (pp. 153–156). Cambridge, MA: MIT Press.

House, L. (1998). *Introductory phonetics and phonology.* Mahwah, NJ: Lawrence Erlbaum.

Ingram, D. (1981). *Procedures for the phonological analysis of children's language*. Baltimore, MD: University Park Press.

Jakobson, R. (1941). *Child language, aphasia and phonological universals*. The Hague & Paris, France: Mouton.

Jakobson, R., Gunnar, C., Fant, M., & Halle, M. (1952). Preliminaries to speech analysis: The distinctive features and their correlates. *Technical Report 13*. Cambridge, MA: Acoustics Laboratory, MIT.

Jakobson, R. (1968). *Phonology in relation to phonetics*. Amsterdam: North-Holland Publishing Co.

Kent, R. (1998). Normal aspects of articulation. In J.E. Bernthal & N.W. Bankson (Eds.), *Articulation and phonological disorders* (4th ed., pp. 1–62).

Kent, R., & Murray, A. (1982). Acoustic features of infant vocalic utterances at 3, 6, and 9 months. *Journal of the Acoustical Society of America, 72*(2), 353–364.

Kent, R., & Read, C. (2002). *The acoustic analysis of speech* (2nd ed.). Ablany, NY: Thomson Learning.

Ladefoged, P. (2005). *Vowels and consonants.* Oxford, UK: Blackwell.

Ladefoged, P. (2006). *A course in phonetics* (5th ed.). San Francisco, CA: Cengage Learning.

LaPointe, L. (2011). *Aphasia and related neurogenic language disorders* (4th ed.). Stuttgart, Germany: Thieme.

Lonigan, C. J., Burgess, S. R., Anthony, J. L., & Barker, T. A. (1998). Development of phonological sensitivity in two- to five-year-old children. *Journal of Educational Psychology*, 90, 294–311.

MacKay, D. G. (1987). *The organization of perception and action: A theory for language and other cognitive skills.* New York, NY: Springer.

MacKay, I. R., & MacKay, I. R. (1987). *Phonetics: The science of speech production.* Boston, MA: Little, Brown.

Macken, M., & Ferguson, C. A. (1983). Cognitive aspects of phonological development: Model, evidence and issues. In K. E. Nelson (ed.), *Children's language*, 4. Hillsdale, NJ: Lawrence Erlbaum.

Moats, L. C. (1995). The missing foundation in teacher education. *American Educator (Special Issue: Learning to Read: Schoolings First Mission), 19*(2), 9, 43–51.

Mowrer, O.H. (1952). Speech development in the young child: The autism theory of speech development and some clinical applications. *Journal of Speech and Hearing Disorders,* 17: 263–268.

McCarter, P. (1974). The early diffusion of the alphabet. *The Biblical Archaeologist, 37*(3), 54–68.

O'Grady, W., Archibald, J., Aronoff, M. J., & Rees-Miller, J. (2001) *Contemporary linguistics* (4th ed.). Location: Bedford/St. Martin's.

Ohde, R. N., & Sharf, D. J. (1992). *Phonetic analysis of normal and abnormal speech.* New York, NY: Merrill.

Oller, D. K. (1980). The emergence of the sounds of speech in infancy. In G. H. Yeni-Komshian, J. F. Kavanaugh, and C. A. Ferguson (Eds.), *Child phonology, Vol. 1: Production.* New York, NY: Academic Press.

Olmsted, D. (1966). *Achumawi Dictionary.* Berkeley, CA: University of California Press.

Parker, F., & Riley, K. (2010). *Linguistics for non-linguists: A primer with exercises* (5th ed.). Boston, MA: Ally & Bacon.

Peña-Brooks, A., & Hegde, M. N. (2000). *Assessment and treatment of articulation and phonological disorders in children: A dual level text.* Austin, TX: Pro-Ed.

Pennington, M. (2010, June). English language rules governing primary stress. (Web log post). Pennington Publishing Blog. Retrieved from http://blog.penningtonpublishing.com/reading/ten-english-accent-rules/.

Perkins, W., & Kent, R. (1986). *Functional anatomy of speech, language and hearing: A primer.* San Diego, CA: College-Hill Press.

Poole, I. (1934). Genetic development of articulation of consonant sounds in speech. *Elementary English Review,* 2, 159–161.

Prather, E., Hendrick, D., & Kern, C. (1975). Articulation development in children aged two to four years. *Journal of Speech and Hearing Disorders, 40*, 179–191.

Raphael, L. J., Borden, G. J., & Harris, K. S. (2007). *Speech science primer: Physiology, acoustics, and perception of speech*. Lipponcott Williams & Wilkins.

Robertson, C., & Salter, W. (1997). *The phonological awareness test (PAT).* East Moline, IL: Linguisystems.

Schwartz, R. G., & Leonard, L.B. (1982). Do children pick and choose? An examination of phonological selection and avoidance in early lexical acquisition. *Journal of Child Language*, 9, 319–336.

Seikel, J. A., Drumright, D. G., & Seikel, P. (2013). *Essentials of anatomy & physiology for communication disorders.* Clifton Park, NY: Delmar Cengage Learning.

Shipley, K., and McAfee, J. (1998) *Assessment in speech language pathology: A resource manual* (2nd ed.). San Diego, CA: Singular Publishing Group.

Shriberg, L. D., & Kent, R.D. (1995). *Clinical phonetics* (2nd ed.). Boston, MA: Allyn & Bacon.

Shriberg, L. D., & Kent, R. D. (2013). *Clinical phonetics*. Boston, MA: Pearson Education.

Shriberg, L. D., & Kwiatkowski, J. (1980). *Natural process analysis: A procedure for phonological analysis of continuous speech samples*. New York, NY: Wiley.

Singh, S., & Singh, K. S. (2006). *Phonetics, principles and practices*. San Diego: Plural Publishing.

Skinner, B. F. (1953). *Science and human behavior*. New York, NY: Simon & Schuster.

Small, L. H. (2005). *Fundamentals of phonetics: A practical guide for students*. Boston, MA: Pearson/Allyn and Bacon.

Stampe, D. (1969). The acquisition of phonemic representation. *Proceedings of the Fifth Regional Meeting of the Chicago Linguistic Society.*

Stoel-Gammon, C., & Dunn, C. (1985). *Normal and disordered phonology in children.* Location: University Park Press.

Templin, M. C. (1957). Certain language skills in children, their development and interrelationships. *Institute of Child Welfare, Monograph Series*, 26. Minneapolis: University of Minnesota Press.

Van Riper, C., & Erickson, R. (1996). *Speech correction: An introduction to speech pathology and audiology* (9th ed). Boston, MA: Allyn & Bacon

Van Riper, C., & Smith, D. E. (1992). *An introduction to general American phonetics*. Prospect Heights, IL: Waveland Press.

Van Riper, C.G. & Smith, D.E. (1979). *An Introduction to general American phonetics* (2nd ed.). Prospect Heights, IL: Waveland Press.

Van Riper, C.G., & Smith, D.E. (1992). *An Introduction to general American phonetics* (3rd ed.). Prospect Heights, IL: Waveland Press.

Vihman, M. M. (1996). *Phonological development.* Oxford, UK: Blackwell

Waterson, N. (1970). Some speech forms of an English child: A phonological study. *Transactions of the Philological Society*, 1–24.

Werker, J. F., & Polka, L. (1993). The ontogeny and developmental significance of language-specific phonetic perception. *NATO ASI Series, 69*, 275–288.

West, R. W., & Kantner, C. E. (1941). *Phonetics: An introduction to the principles of phonetic science from the point of view of English speech.* London, UK: Harper & Brothers.

West, R. W., & Kantner, C.E. (1941). *Phonetics: An introduction to the principles of phonetic science from the point of view of English speech.* New York; London: Harper & Brothers.

Yavas, M. S. (2006). *Applied English phonology*. Malden, MA: Blackwell.

APPENDIX

Distinctive Features: Stops

Stops	/p/	/b/	/t/	/d/	/k/	/g/
Obstruent						
Sonorant						
Consonantal						
Vocalic						
Continuant						
Interrupted						
Anterior						
Back						
Strident						
Coronal						
Lateral						
Rounded						

(*Continued*)

Labial						
Nasal						
Voice						
Stops	/p/	/b/	/t/	/d/	/k/	/g/

Distinctive Features: Fricatives

Fricatives	/f/	/v/	/θ/	/ð/	/s/	/z/	/ʃ/	/ʒ/	/h/
Obstruent									
Sonorant									
Consonantal									
Vocalic									
Continuant									
Interrupted									
Anterior									

Back									
Strident									
Coronal									
Lateral									
Rounded									
Labial									
Nasal									
Voice									
Fricatives									

Obstruents	/p/	/b/	/t/	/d/	/k/	/g/	/f/	/v/	/θ/	/ð/	/s/	/z/	/ʃ/	/ʒ/	/h/	/ʧ/	/ʤ/
Obstruent																	
Sonorant																	
Consonantal																	
Vocalic																	
Continuant																	
Interrupted																	
Anterior																	
Back																	
Strident																	
Coronal																	
Lateral																	
Rounded																	

Labial																	
Nasal																	
Voice																	
Obstruents																	

Distinctive Features: Sonorants

Sonorants	/w/	/j/	/l/	/r/	/m/	/n/	/ŋ/
Obstruent							
Sonorant							
Consonantal							
Vocalic							
Continuant							
Interrupted							
Anterior							

(*Continued*)

Back							
Strident							
Coronal							
Lateral							
Rounded							
Labial							
Nasal							
Voice							
Sonorants							

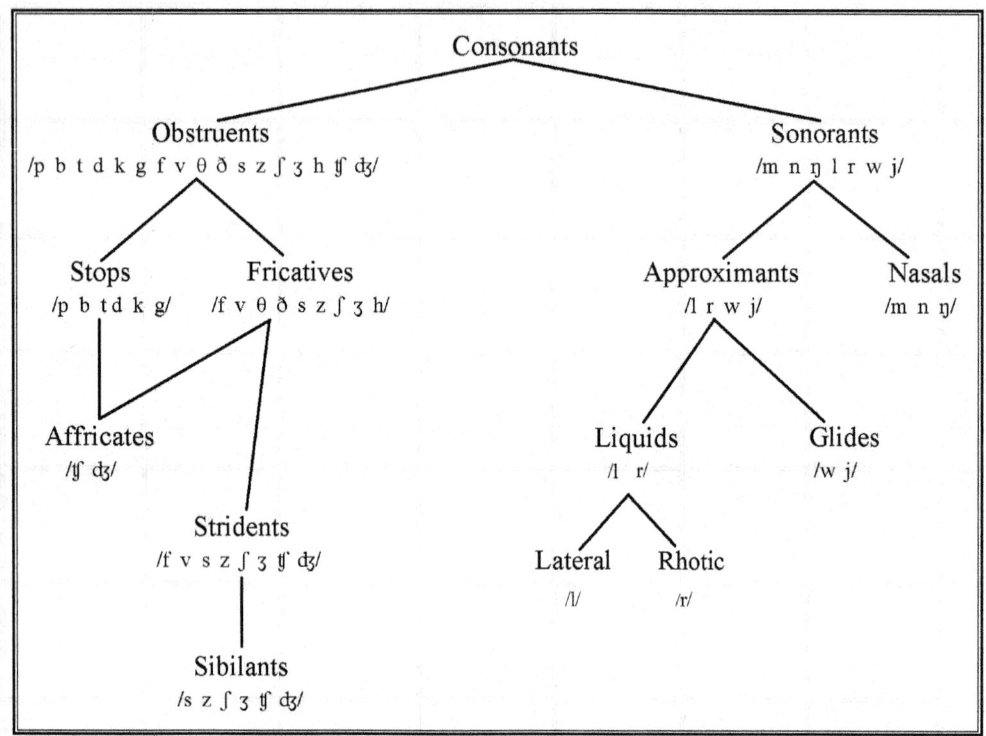

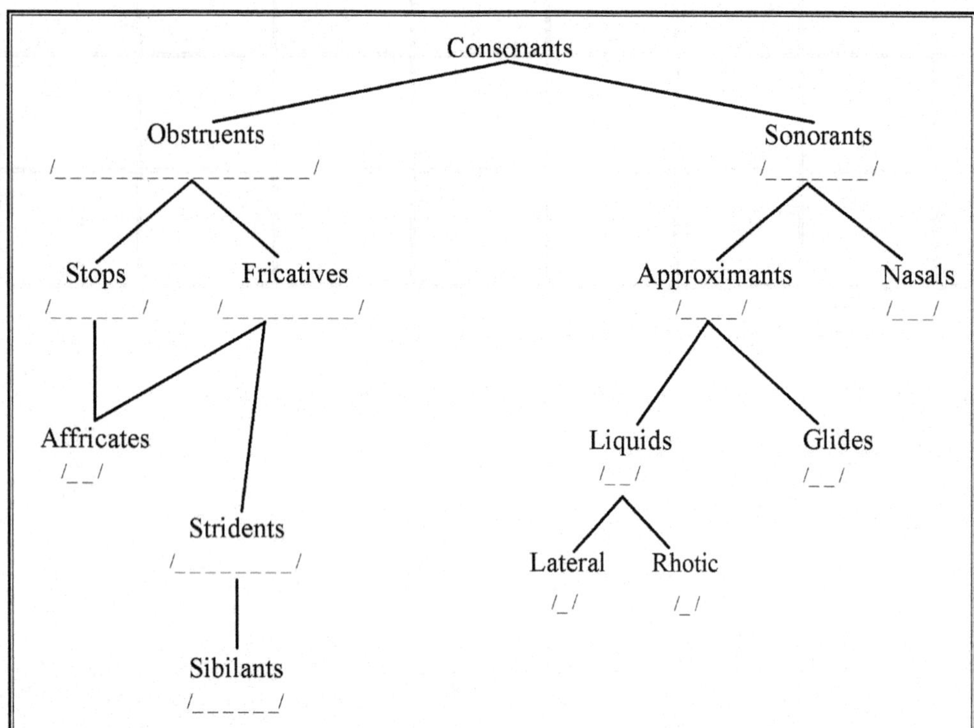

Fig. 6.1a-b: Consonant Tree

ANSWER KEY

CHAPTER 1

Exercise 1.1 Identify the silent graphemes:

Wrap *w*	Wednesday *d*	Lamb *b*	Thumb *b*
Subtle *b*	Gnome *g*	Psychic *p*	Receipt *t*
Autumn *n*	Assign *g*	Cologne *g*	Knee *k*
Honest *h*	Knife *k*	Yolk *l*	Island *s*
Ballet *t*	Gnat *g*	Answer *s*	Psalm *p*

Exercise 1.2 Identify the number of graphemes and phonemes in the following words:

Orthographic	# of G	# of P	Orthographic	# of G	# of P
Chip	4	3	Sawed	5	3
Hat	3	3	Mix	3	4
Clap	4	4	Bring	5	4
Face	4	3	Write	5	3

(*Continued*)

Run	3	3	Know	4	2
Does	4	3	Loose	5	3
Stash	5	4	Throat	6	4
Wrinkle	7	5	Tea	3	2
That	4	3	Thorough	8	4
Back	4	3	Quack	5	4

Exercise 1.3 Identify the number of morphemes in the following words:

Orthographic	Morphemes	Number	Orthographic	Morphemes	Number
Bats	Bat-s	2	Slices	Slice-s	2
Ran	Ran	1	Boyishness	Boy-ish-ness	3
Walking	Walk-ing	2	Downtown	Down-town	2
It's	It-'s	2	Grapes	Grape-s	2
Higher	High-er	2	Gentleman	Gentle-man	2

Around	Around	1	Water	Water	1
Rebound	Re-bound	2	Drawing	Draw-ing	2
Basketball	Basket-ball	2	Paints	Paint-s	2
Unhappiest	Un-happi-est	3	Jeff's	Jeff-'s	2
Dogs	Dog-s	2	Haircut	Hair-cut	2

Exercise 1.4 Underline the *cluster* in the following words:

Splash	Squid	Spill	Cluster	Black
Desk	Swing	Plate	Spring	Stripe
Spray	Plaster	Spots	Clasp	Blast
Queen	Mask	Chest	Glow	Scallop

Exercise 1.5 Identify the digraph in each of the following words:

hush	**sh**	ships	**sh**
growth	**th**	switch	**tch**
thrush	**th, sh**	philosophy	**ph**
church	**ch**	laughing	**gh**
trash	**sh**	swing	**ng**
phone	**ph**	shout	**sh**
beach	**ch**	digraph	**ph**
pocket	**ck**	whale	**wh**
which	**wh, ch**	mouth	**th**
clock	**ck**	bridge	**dg**

Exercise 1.6 Identify if each consonant is prevocalic, intervocalic, or postvocalic:

Orthographic Word	Prevocalic	Intervocalic	Postvocalic
ballet	b	l	
carrot	**k**	**r**	**t**
hope	**h**		**p**
button	**b**	**t**	**n**
colon	**k**	**l**	**n**
narrow	**n**	**r**	
dog	**d**		**g**
wagon	**w**	**g**	**n**
boat	**b**		**t**
cook	**k**		**k**

Exercise 1.7 Identify the number of syllables in each of the following words:

Orthographic	Identify syllables	Number of Syllables
popcorn	pop-corn	2
night	**night**	**1**
you	**You**	**1**
thinking	**Think-ing**	**2**
football	**Foot-ball**	**2**
elements	**El-e-ments**	**3**
tour	**Tour**	**1**
directions	**di-rec-tions**	**3**
super	**Su-per**	**2**
jargon	**Jar-gon**	**2**
superstition	**Su-per-sti-tion**	**4**
aardvark	**Aard-vark**	**2**

trampoline	**Tramp-o-line**	**3**
dig	**Dig**	**1**
segments	**Seg-ments**	**2**
earlobe	**Ear-lobe**	**2**
scramble	**Scram-ble**	**2**
down	**down**	**1**
up	**up**	**1**
I	**I**	**1**

CHAPTER 3

Exercise 3.1 Add a rhyming word to each example:

Orthographic	IPA
blue	/blu/
clue	/klu/

you	**/ju/**
mitt	/mɪt/
pit	/pɪt/
sit	/sɪt/
cat	/kæt/
hat	/hæt/
bat	**/bæt/**
game	/gem/
name	/nem/
fame	**/fem/**
flew	/flu/
through	/θru/
grew	**/gru/**

CHAPTER 4

Exercise 4.1 Transcribe the following words containing /i/.

1. beam	/bim/	6. keen	/kin/
2. dean	/din/	7. lean	/lin/
3. ease	/iz/	8. heat	/hit/
4. free	/fri /	9. peace	/pis/
5. glee	/gli/	10. greet	/grit/

Exercise 4.2 Identify the following words:

1. /fli/	flee	6. /lig/	league
2. /drim/	dream	7. /mik/	meek
3. /krip/	creep	8. /did/	deed
4. /bist/	beast	9. /grin/	green
5. /lif/	leaf	10. /hip/	heap

Exercise 4.3 Transcribe the following words containing /ɪ/:

1. bid	/bɪd	6. him	/hɪm/
2. tin	/tɪn/	7. lip	/lɪp/
3. pig	/pɪg/	8. kid	/kɪd/
4. dim	/dɪm/	9. fig	/fɪg/
5. lid	/lɪd/	10. fin	/fɪn/

Exercise 4.4 Identify the following words:

1. /bɪg/	**big**	6. /dɪd/	**did**
2. /pɪn/	**pin**	7. /fɪn/	**fin**
3. /tɪp/	**tip**	8. /lɪd/	**lid**
4. /hɪt/	**hit**	9. /grɪn/	**grin**
5. /dɪg/	**dig**	10. /hɪp/	**hip**

Exercise 4.5 Differentiate /i/ and /ɪ/ by circling the vowel in each word:

evil	**/i/**	/ɪ/	lid	/i/	**/ɪ/**
hymn	/i/	**/ɪ/**	seam	**/i/**	/ɪ/
gym	/i/	**/ɪ/**	these	**/i/**	/ɪ/
ski	**/i/**	/ɪ/	give	/i/	**/ɪ/**
built	/i/	**/ɪ/**	eve	**/i/**	/ɪ/
tea	**/i/**	/ɪ/	list	/i/	**/ɪ/**
seat	**/i/**	/ɪ/	sieve	/i/	/ɪ/
ship	/i/	**/ɪ/**	feast	**/i/**	/ɪ/
seek	**/i/**	/ɪ/	skip	/i/	**/ɪ/**
rich	/i/	**/ɪ/**	risk	/i/	**/ɪ/**

Exercise 4.6 Transcribe the following words containing /e/:

1. bait	**/bet/**	6. Gain	**/gen/**
2. dane	**/den/**	7. braid	**/bred/**
3. train	**/tren/**	8. hay	**/he/**
4. brain	**/bren/**	9. place	**/ples/**
5. fain	**/fen/**	10. aim	**/em/**

Exercise 4.7 Identify the following words:

1. /ren/	**rain**	6. /wet/	**wait**
2. /dren/	**drain**	7. /fes/	**face**
3. /plen/	**plain, plane**	8. /pest/	**paste**
4. /le/	**lay, lei**	9. /gren/	**grain**
5. /wev/	**wave**	10. /greps/	**grapes**

Exercise 4.8 Transcribe the following words containing /ɛ/:

1. beg	**/bɛg/**	6. desk	**/dɛsk/**
2. hen	**/hɛn/**	7. pest	**/pɛst/**
3. egg	**/ɛg/**	8. head	**/hɛd/**
4. wept	**/wɛpt/**	9. guest	**/gɛst/**
5. leg	**/lɛg/**	10. guess	**/gɛs/**

Exercise 4.9 Identify the following words:

1. /ɛlf/	**elf**	6. /lɛft/	**left**
2. /frɛnd/	**friend**	7. /ɛnd/	**end**
3. /dɛt/	**debt**	8. /dɛd/	**dead**
4. /nɛt/	**knelt**	9. /pɛn/	**pen**
5. /pɛg/	**peg**	10. /stɛpt/	**stepped**

Exercise 4.10 Circle the vowel in each word:

1.	wet	**/ɛ/**	/ɪ/	wit	/ɛ/	**/ɪ/**
2.	ten	**/ɛ/**	/ɪ/	tin	/ɛ/	**/ɪ/**
3.	beg	**/ɛ/**	/ɪ/	big	/ɛ/	**/ɪ/**
4.	mitt	/ɛ/	**/ɪ/**	met	**/ɛ/**	/ɪ/
5.	bed	**/ɛ/**	/ɪ/	bid	/ɛ/	**/ɪ/**
6.	set	**/ɛ/**	/ɪ/	sit	/ɛ/	**/ɪ/**
7.	net	**/ɛ/**	/ɪ/	knit	/ɛ/	**/ɪ/**
8.	bit	/ɛ/	**/ɪ/**	bet	**/ɛ/**	/ɪ/
9.	lit	/ɛ/	**/ɪ/**	let	**/ɛ/**	/ɪ/
10.	den	**/ɛ/**	/ɪ/	din	/ɛ/	**/ɪ/**

Exercise 4.11 Transcribe the following words containing /æ/:

1. ask	**/æsk/**	6. gas	**/gæs/**
2. zap	**/zæp/**	7. bag	**/bæg/**
3. hat	**/hæt/**	8. dab	**/dæb/**
4. sad	**/sæd/**	9. map	**/mæp/**
5. fat	**/fæt/**	10. lab	**/læb/**

Exercise 4.12 Identify the following words:

1. /bæs/	**bass**	6. /glæd/	**glad**
2. /æt/	**at**	7. /mæs/	**mass**
3. /læf/	**laugh**	8. /læst/	**last**
4. /kæf/	**calf**	9. /snæp/	**snap**
5. /hæz/	**has**	10. /hæv/	**have**

Exercise 4.13 Transcribe the front vowels in the following words:

1. that	/æ/	7. pat	/æ/
2. mate	/e/	8. head	/ɛ/
3. jet	/ɛ/	9. pin	/ɪ/
4. meet	/i/	10. beach	/i/
5. nap	/æ/	11. day	/e/
6. Roy	/ɔɪ/	12. beige	/e/

13. peach	/i/	27. late	/e/
14. pain	/e/	28. Rate	/e/
15. chief	/i/	29. pet	/ɛ/
16. his	/ɪ/	30. feed	/i/
17. tease	/i/	31. debt	/ɛ/
18. rinse	/ɪ/	32. leap	/i/
19. knelt	/ɛ/	33. fate	/e/
20. lean	/i/	34. date	/e/
21. each	/i/	35. bat	/æ/
22. mat	/æ/	36. black	/æ/
23. big	/ɪ/	37. heave	/i/
24. age	/e/	38. swim	/ɪ/
25. gaze	/e/	39. speck	/ɛ/
26. preach	/i/	40. lain	/e/

Exercise 4.14 Transcribe the following words containing /u/;

1. moo	/mu/	6. two	/tu/
2. flute	/flut/	7. zoo	/zu/
3. prune	/prun/	8. tune	/tun/
4. blew	/blu/	9. spoon	/spun/
5. sue	/su/	10. plume	/plum/

Exercise 4.15 Identify the following words:

1. /flu/	**flu, flew**	6. /gus/	**goose**
2. /dru/	**drew**	7. /sut/	**suit**
3. /muv/	**move**	8. /gru/	**grew**
4. /but/	**boot**	9. /grum/	**groom**
5. /brum/	**broom**	10. /hu/	**who**

Exercise 4.16 Transcribe the following words containing /ʊ/:

1. book	**/bʊk/**	6. soot	**/sʊt/**
2. look	**/lʊk/**	7. foot	**/fʊt/**
3. good	**/gʊd/**	8. wool	**/wʊl/**
4. wood	**/wʊd/**	9. put	**/pʊt/**
5. cook	**/kʊk/**	10. wolf	**/wʊlf/**

Exercise 4.17 Identify the following words:

1. /pʊl/	**pull**	6. /krʊk/	**crook**
2. /kʊd/	**could**	7. /tʊk/	**took**
3. /bʊks/	**books**	8. /brʊk/	**brook**
4. /wʊdz/	**woods**	9. /fʊt/	**foot**
5. /lʊkt/	**looked**	10. /hʊd/	**hood**

Exercise 4.18 Transcribe the following words containing /o/:

1. toad	/tod/	6. told	/told/
2. bone	/bon/	7. sold	/sold/
3. rode	/rod/	8. row	/ro/
4. beau	/bo/	9. slow	/slo/
5. post	/post/	10. mode	/mod/

Exercise 4.19 Identify the following words:

1. /flo/	flow	6. /logo/	logo
2. /kro/	crow	7. /kom/	comb
3. /bo/	beau, bow	8. /dop/	dope
4. /bost/	boast	9. /gro/	grow
5. /lon/	loan	10. /hop/	hope

Exercise 4.20 Transcribe the following words containing /ɔ/:

1. law	/lɔ/	6. off	/ɔf/
2. flaw	/flɔ/	7. raw	/rɔ/
3. spawn	/spɔn/	8. paw	/pɔ/
4. drawn	/drɔn/	9. caught	/kɔt/
5. scrawl	/skrɔl/	10. salt	/sɔlt/

Exercise 4.21 Identify the following words:

1. /sɔ/	**saw**	6. /lɔ/	**law**
2. /lɔn/	**lawn**	7. /kɔzd/	**caused**
3. /krɔl/	**crawl**	8. /frɔd/	**fraud**
4. /pɔn/	**pawn**	9. /fɔlt/	**fault**
5. /skɔld/	**scald**	10. /hɔnt/	**haunt**

Exercise 4.22 Transcribe the following words containing /*ɑ*/:

1. hot	**/hɑt/**	6. blot	**/blɑt/**
2. trot	**/trɑt/**	7. slot	**/slɑt/**
3. lot	**/lɑt/**	8. pot	**/pɑt/**
4. knot	**/nɑt/**	9. dot	**/dɑt/**
5. got	**/gɑt/**	10. swap	**/swɑp/**

Exercise 4.23 Identify the following words:

1. /tɑps/	**tops**	6. /drɑp /	**drop**
2. /slɑb /	**slob**	7. /bɑks /	**box**
3. /klɑk /	**clock**	8. /pɑp/	**pop**
4. /fɑks /	**fox**	9. /mɑm /	**mom**
5./ nɑks /	**knocks**	10. /spɑ/	**spa**

Exercise 4.24 Differentiating /ɔ/ and /ɑ/ in minimal pairs. Circle the vowel in each word:

1.	hawk	**(/ɔ/)**	/ɑ/	hock	/ɔ/	**(/ɑ/)**
2.	Don	/ɔ/	**(/ɑ/)**	dawn	**(/ɔ/)**	/ɑ/
3.	odd	/ɔ/	**(/ɑ/)**	awed	**(/ɔ/)**	/ɑ/
4.	raw	**(/ɔ/)**	/ɑ/	rah	/ɔ/	**(/ɑ/)**
5.	cot	/ɔ/	**(/ɑ/)**	caught	**(/ɔ/)**	/ɑ/
6.	sought	**(/ɔ/)**	/ɑ/	sot	/ɔ/	**(/ɑ/)**

Exercise 4.25 Transcribe the back vowels in the following words:

1. ooze	/u/	21. cot	/ɑ/
2. caught	/ɔ/	22. law	/ɔ/
3. dog	/ɑ/	23. fought	/ɔ/
4. hope	/o/	24. toe	/o/
5. nope	/o/	25. shoot	/u/
6. took	/ʊ/	26. hot	/ɑ/
7. boat	/o/	27. all	/ɔ/
8. cook	/ʊ/	28. pull	/ʊ/
9. grew	/u/	29. snooze	/u/
10. soup	/u/	30. shook	/ʊ/
11. vote	/o/	31. foot	/ʊ/
12. brook	/ʊ/	32. tube	/u/
13. put	/ʊ/	33. pause	/ɔ/

(*Continued*)

14. draw	/ɔ/	34. hook	/ʊ/
15. true	/u/	35. drop	/ɑ/
16. rope	/o/	36. rose	/o/
17. straw	/ɔ/	37. group	/u/
18. book	/ʊ/	38. scald	/ɔ/
19. pop	/ɑ/	39. spot	/ɑ/
20. flute	/u/	40. clue	/u/

Exercise 4.26 Transcribe the following words, which contain Front and Back vowels:

Front		Back	
1. bee	/bi/	11. boo	/bu/
2. pit	/pɪt/	12. put	/pʊt/
3. came	/kem/	13. comb	/kom/
4. pen	/pɛn/	14. pawn	/pɔn/
5. pat	/pæt/	15. pot	/pɑt/
6. key	/ki/	16. coo	/ku/
7. fit	/fIt/	17. foot	/fʊt/
8. gate	/get/	18. goat	/got/
9. heck	/hɛk/	19. hawk	/hɔk/
10. slab	/slæb/	20. slob	/slɑb/

Exercise 4.27 Transcribe the following words containing /ʌ/:

1. bum	**/bʌm/**	6. mug	**/mʌg/**
2. dun	**/dʌn/**	7. sub	**/sʌb/**
3. cut	**/kʌt/**	8. hut	**/hʌt/**
4. bug	**/bʌg/**	9. dug	**/dʌg/**
5. gun	**/gʌn/**	10. bus	**/bʌs/**

Exercise 4.28 Read the phonetic symbols to identify the following words:

1. /flʌd/	**flood**	6. /lʌg/	**lug**
2. /drʌm/	**drum**	7. /mʌk/	**muck**
3. /kʌp/	**cup**	8. /mʌt/	**mutt**
4. /bʌst/	**bust**	9. /sʌn/	**sun**
5. /hʌg/	**hug**	10. /hʌmp/	**hump**

Exercise 4.29 Transcribe the following words containing /ə/ in the first syllable, which is unstressed:

1. away	**/əwe/**
2. alone	**/əlon/**
3. again	**/əgɛn/**
4. across	**/əkrɔs/**

Exercise 4.30 Transcribe the following words containing /ə/ in the second syllable which is unstressed:

1. sofa	/sofə/
2. soda	/sodə/
3. coma	/komə/
4. gallop	/gæləp/
5. okra	/okrə/

Exercise 4.31 Transcribe the following words containing /ɝ/:

Word	Transcription	Word	Transcription
1. burn	/bɝn/	6. girl	/gɝl/
2. first	/fɝst/	7. twirl	/twɝl/
3. irk	/ɝk/	8. fur	/fɝ/
4. sir	/sɝ/	9. purr	/pɝ/
5. dirt	/dɝt/	10. worm	/wɝm/

Exercise 4.32 Read the phonetic symbols to identify the following words:

1. /pɝk/	perk	6. /stɝ/	stir
2. /skɝt/	skirt	7. /kɝb/	curb
3. /wɝk/	work	8. /sɝv/	serve
4. /bɝst/	burst	9. /nɝd/	nerd
5./ lɝk/	lurk	10. /kɝs/	curse

Exercise 4.33 Transcribe the following words containing /ɚ/:

1. sister	/sɪstɚ/
2. butter	/bətɚ/
3. bitter	/bɪtɚ/
4. under	/ʌndɚ/
5. over	/ovɚ/

Exercise 4.34 Name each vowel:

1. Low, Front	æ
2. Low-mid, Central	ʌ
3. High, Back	u
4. High-mid, Front	ɪ
5. Mid-central, Tense, Rounded	ɝ
6. Low-mid, Back	ɔ
7. High, Front	i
8. Unstressed Rhotic	ɚ
9. Mid, Front	e
10. Mid, Back	o
11. Unstressed Neutral	ə
12. Low, Back	ɑ
13. Low-mid, Front	ɛ
14. Low, Front	æ

Exercise 4.35 Transcribe all the vowels in the following words:

1. August	/ɔ, ə/
2. panda	/æ, ə/
3. delta	/ɛ, ə/
4. necessary	/ɛ, ə, ɛr, i/
5. attack	/ə, æ/
6. often	/ɔ, ɪ/
7. alert	/ə, ɝ/
8. cobra	/o, ə/
9. column	/ɑ, ə/
10. suffice	/ə, aɪ/

Exercise 4.36 Transcribe the front, central, and back vowels heard in the following words:

	Front		Central		Back	
1.	bead	/i/	bird	/ɝ/	bode	/o/
2.	pit	/ɪ/	putt	/ʌ/	put	/ʊ/
3.	pain	/e/	pun	/ʌ/	pawn	/ɔ/
4.	peg	/ɛ/	pug	/ʌ/	pog	/ɑ/
5.	cat	/æ/	curt	/ɝ/	caught	/ɔ/
6.	mat	/æ/	mutt	/ʌ/	moat	/o/
7.	ten	/ɛ/	turn	/ɝ/	tune	/u/
8.	gain	/e/	gun	/ʌ/	goon	/u/
9.	fin	/ɪ/	fun	/ʌ/	phone	/o/
10.	teen	/i/	ton	/ʌ/	tone	/o/

Exercise 4.37 Transcribe the following words containing /ɔɪ/:

1. boy	/bɔɪ/
2. soy	/sɔɪ/
3. toy	/tɔɪ/
4. voice	/vɔɪs/
5. spoil	/spɔɪl/

Exercise 4.38 Transcribe the following words containing /aʊ/:

1. cow	/kaʊ/
2. foul	/faʊl/
3. now	/naʊ/
4. doubt	/daʊt/
5. wow	/waʊ/

Exercise 4.39 Transcribe the following words containing /aɪ/:

1. knife	/naɪf/
2. tight	/taɪt/
3. might	/maɪt/
4. life	/laɪf/
5. strife	/straɪf/

Exercise 4.40 Transcribe the following words containing /ju/:

1. muse	/mjuz/
2. fuze	/fjuz/
3. fume	/fjum/
4. used	/juzd/
5. few	/fju/

Exercise 4.41 Transcribe the diphthongs in the following words:

1. how	/aʊ/	7. bite	/aɪ/
2. mine	/aɪ/	8. crown	/aʊ/
3. joy	/ɔɪ/	9. use	/ju/
4. high	/aɪ/	10. toy	/ɔɪ/
5. now	/aʊ/	11. dice	/aɪ/
6. Roy	/ɔɪ/	12. cloud	/aʊ/
13. hound	/aʊ/	27. ouch	/aʊ/
14. pie	/aɪ/	28. time	/aɪ/
15. prowl	/aʊ/	29. sigh	/aɪ/
16. I	/aɪ/	30. outside	/aʊ/, /aɪ/
17. ointment	/ɔɪ/	31. house	/aʊ/
18. choice	/ɔɪ/	32. lie	/aɪ/
19. plough	/aʊ/	33. about	/aʊ/
20.oil	/ɔɪ/	34. cute	/ju/
21. oyster	/ɔɪ/	35. poise	/ɔɪ/

22. eyes	/aɪ/	36. ounce	/aʊ/
23. you	/ju/	37. boy	/ɔɪ/
24. ice	/aɪ/	38. avoid	/ɔɪ/
25. owl	/aʊ/	39. Hide	/aɪ/
26. mouse	/aʊ/	40. beauty	/ju/

Exercise 4.42 Transcribe the rhotic diphthongs and triphthongs in the following words:

1. square	/ɛr/	7. hour	/aʊr/
2. dire	/aɪr/	8. tire	/aɪr/
3. board	/ɔr/	9. pier	/ɪr/
4. hair	/ɛr/	10. arm	/ɑr/
5. bear	/ɛr/	11. deer	/ɪr/
6. tore	/ɔr/	12. four	/ɔr/
13. store	/ɔr/	27. our	/aʊr/
14. stare	/ɛr/	28. heir	/ɛr/
15. pear	/ɛr/	29. clear	/ɪr/
16. choir	/aɪr/	30. tier	/ɪr/
17. pork	/ɔr/	31. dare	/ɛr/
18. mare	/ɛr/	32. mar	/ɑr/
19. beer	/ɪr/	33. star	/ɑr/
20. cork	/ɔr/	34. mire	/aɪr/
21. Tour	/ʊr/	35. pour	/ʊr/

(*Continued*)

22. ear	/ɪr/	36. park	/ɑr/
23. card	/ɑr/	37. pier	/ɪr/
24. beard	/ɪr/	38. dare	/ɛr/
25. fear	/ɪr/	39. fair	/ɛr/
26. barn	/ɑr/	40. glare	/ɛr/

CHAPTER 5

Exercise 5.1 Based on what you have learned about stress, underline the syllable that receives primary stress in the following words:

expert	demand	July
attempt	information	water
amount	composer	expensive
rescue	country	reply
defense	argue	gorilla
remainder	system	central
mental	effect	remember
detective	research	increase

demand	December	machine
control	number	problem
departure	complain	engine
disease	emotion	another
eclipse	barracuda	accommodation
canal	expect	presentation

CHAPTER 7

Exercise 7.1 Identify the following words:

1. /ʌpɚ/	upper	16. /pop/	pope
2. /bʌd/	bud	17. /pækt/	packed
3. /pʌp/	pup	18. /dip/	deep
4. /pɑp/	pop	19. /tep/	tape
5. /pæd/	pad	20. /bip/	beep
6. /kʌt/	cut	21. /gʌt/	gut
7. /bæg/	bag	22. /tept/	taped
8. /dɑkt/	docked	23. /detə/	data
9. /totɛd/	totted	24. /pɪki/	picky
10. /tæki/	tacky	25. /pɝki/	perky

(*Continued*)

11. /kot/	coat	26. /botɚ/	boater
12. /bɑbi/	Bobby	27. /kæbi/	cabbie
13. /bʌtɚ/	butter	28. /ɔdæpt/	adapt
14. /kæt/	cat	29. /gaɪ/	guy
15. /daɪd/	died	30. /kʌp/	cup

Exercise 7.2 Transcribe the following words:

1. ape	/ep/	16. but	/bʌt/
2. peep	/pip/	17. bed	/bɛd/
3. beat	/bit/	18. pet	/pɛt/
4. back	/bæk/	19. Abe	/eb/
5. good	/gʊd/	20. puppet	/pʌpɛt/
6. tick	/tɪk/	21. cookie	/kʊki/
7. guppy	/gʌpi/	22. doctor	/dɑktɚ/
8. paperback	/pepɚbæk/	23. pack	/pæk/
9. pucker	/pʌkɚ/	24. cape	/kep/
10. dog	/dɑg/	25. taupe	/top/
11. took	/tʊk/	26.putt	/pʌt/
12. bigger	/bɪgɚ/	27. bagboy	/bægbɔɪ/
13. dagger	/dægɚ/	28. dirty	/dɝti/
14. debate	/dəbet/	29. ticket	/tɪkɛt/
15. attack	/ətæk/	30. toad	/tod/

Exercise 7.4

Down		Across	
1. under	/ʌndɚ/	1. puddle	/pʌdl̩/
2. back	/bæk/	2. tab	/tæb/
		3. keg	/kɛg/

Exercise 7.5 Circle whether the voicing of the two words is same or different:

Words:		Voicing: Same or Different
1. thy	thigh	D
2. bath	bathe	D
3. thunder	thirsty	S
4. these	thumb	D
5. thin	third	S
6. with	wither	D
7. smooth	wreath	D
8. breathe	breath	D
9. soothe	south	D
10. myth	mouth	S
11. either	nothing	D
12. leather	lethal	D
13. sympathy	authentic	S

(*Continued*)

14. gather	mother	S
15. worthy	breathy	D
16. farther	father	S
17. teeth	teethe	D

Exercise 7.6 Identify the following words:

1. /tuθ/	tooth	16. /ʃʊgɚ/	sugar
2. /sɪti/	city	17. /sɪzɚz/	scissors
3. /sʌpɚ/	supper	18. /ʃɑk/	shock
4. /fɪʃ/	fish	19. /sit/	seat
5. /kæʃ/	cash	20. /hæθ/	hath
6. /dɪʃɛz/	dishes	21. /kæst/	cast
7. /sɑk/	sock	22. /æʒɚ/	azure
8. /ʃʌks/	shucks	23. /hʌʃt/	hushed
9. /pæst/	past	24. /skɝt/	skirt
10./fɪzd/	fizzed	25. /ʃaʊt/	shout
11. /ʃɝt/	shirt	26. /ðʌs/	thus
12. /huz/	whose	27. /vɔɪs/	voice
13. /bɑðɚ/	bother	28. /ʃɛd/	shed
14. /vaɪzɚ/	visor	29. /ʃu/	shoe
15. /ʃip/	sheep	30. /fɑks/	fox

Exercise 7.7 Transcribe the following words:

1. five	/faɪv/	4. Bob's	/bɑbz/
2. tease	/tiz/	5. huff	/hʌf/
3. zoo	/zu/	6. oars	/ɔrz/
7. high	/haɪ/	19. zigzag	/zɪgzæg/
8. thigh	/θaɪ/	20. shaves	/ʃevz/
9. theft	/θɛft/	21. hat	/hæt/
10. sad	/sæd/	22. tough	/tʌf/
11. vase	/ves/	23. thumb	/θʌm/
12. thought	/θɑt/	24. heft	/hɛft/
13. vote	/vot/	25. veto	/vito/
14. fate	/fet/	26. have	/hæv/
15. soap	/sop/	27. these	/ðiz/
16. zip	/zɪp/	28. dashes	/dæʃɛz/
17. hers	/hɝz/	29. beige	/beʒ/
18. eyes	/aɪz/	30. cost	/kɑst/

Exercise 7.8 Identify what is wrong with the following words. If the word is correct, write "ok"; if the word is incorrect, correct it:

1. push	/pʊʃ/	6. /of/	/ʌv/
2. back	/bæk/	7. off	/ɑf/
3. pop	/pɑp/	8. /ship/	/ʃɪp/

(Continued)

4. soft	/sɑft/	9. /host/	/host/
5. sheep	/ʃip/	10. twos	/tuz/

Exercise 7.9 Identify the following words:

1. / ʤaʊst/	joust	11. /ʤɛst/	jest
2. /ʤe/	Jay	12. /fʌʤ/	fudge
3. /ʤɛsʧɚ/	gesture	13. /ʤʌg/	jug
4. /səʤɛst/	suggest	14. /hæʧɛz/	hatches
5. /bʊʧɚ/	butcher	15. /bɑʧɛz/	batches
6. /fiʧɚ/	feature	16. /əbʤɛkt/	object
7. /ʤæk/	Jack	17. /fɛʧɛz/	fetches
8. /poʧɛz/	poaches	18. /kɛʧəp/	ketchup
9. /tʌʧɛz/	touches	19. /dʌʧɛz/	Dutches
10. /ʤɛt/	jet	20. /piʧɛz/	peaches

Exercise 7.10 Transcribe the following words:

1. chuck	[ʧʌk]	11. choppy	[ʧɑpi]
2. choke	[ʧok]	12. lecture	[lɛkʧɚ]
3. picture	[pɪkʧɚ]	13. chug	[ʧʌg]
4. church	[ʧɝʧ]	14. jig	[ʤɪg]
5. jeer	[ʤɛr]	15. choose	[ʧuz]
6. jiffy	[ʤɪfi]	16. gin	[ʤɪn]
7. chubby	[ʧʌbi]	17. jade	[ʤed]

8. gipsy	[ʤɪpsi]	18. pasture	[pæsʧɚ]
9. jigsaw	[ʤɪgsɔ]	19. jitters	[ʤɪtɚz]
10. chew	[ʧu]	20. chose	[ʧuz]

Exercise 7.12

Down	Across
1. jump [ʤʌmp]	1. judge [ʤʌʤ]
2. change [ʧenʤ]	2. jam [ʤæm]
	3. punch [pʌnʧ]

Exercise 7.13 Transcribe the following words:

1. wood	[wʊd]	11. use	[juz]
2. wake	[wek]	12. wed	[wɛd]
3. wave	[wev]	13. weave	[wiv]
4. witch	[wɪʧ]	14. whack	[wæk]
5. wig	[wɪg]	15. wick	[wɪk]
6. word	[wɝd]	16. yet	[jɛt]
7. wish	[wɪʃ]	17. wet	[wɛt]
8. way	[we]	18. yoke	[jok]
9. wait	[wet]	19. Yea	[je]
10. yeah	[jæ]	20. wow	[waʊ]

Exercise 7.15

Down	Across
1. winning [wɪnɪŋ]	1. watts [wɑts]
2. yacht [jɑt]	2. yawn [jɔn]
3. sweep [swip]	

Exercise 7.16 Identify the following words:

1. /lɑbstɚ/	lobster	6. /ple/	play
2. /stɑrz/	stars	7. /pɪlo/	pillow
3. /lɪpstɪk/	lipstick	8. /pɝLz/	pearls
4. /kənstrʌkt/	construct	9. /rezɔrbæks/	razorbacks
5./dɛltə/	delta	10. /litʃ/	leach

Exercise 7.17 Transcribe the following words:

1. laugh	[læf]	8. allow	[əlaʊ]
2. girl	[gɝL]	9. legalize	[ligəlaɪz]
3. circles	[sɝklɛz]	10. Rick	[rɪk]
4. reword	[riwɝd]	11. lurk	[lɝk]
5. flirtatious	[flɚteʃəs]	12. warrior	[wɔriɚ]
6. reward	[riwɔrd]	13. Jello	[dʒɛlo]
7. lazy	[lezi]	14. repute	[ripjut]

15. wrath	[ræθ]	18. leap	[lip]
16. loop	[lup]	19. robin	[rɑbɪn]
17. bellow	[bɛlo]	20. relish	[rɛlɪʃ]

Exercise 7.19

Down	Across
1. raving [revɪŋ]	1. ramp [ræmp]
2. peel [pɪL]	2. rev [rɛv]
3. roll [roL]	3. ran [ræn]
	4. little [lɪtL̩]

Exercise 7.20 Complete the following exercises, which are designed to help with the transcription of words containing /æ/:

1. Santa	[sæntə]	6. pang	[pæŋ]
2. panda	[pændə]	7. pansy	[pænzi]
3. amber	[æmbɚ]	8. dam	[dæm]
4. Tampa	[tæmpə]	9. tan	[tæn]
5. panic	[pænɪk]	10. family	[fæməli]

Exercise 7.21 Complete the following exercises, which are designed to help with the transcription of words containing nk:

1. prank	[præŋk]	11. pink	[pɪŋk]
2. sank	[sæŋk]	12. rank	[ræŋk]
3. drank	[dræŋk]	13. tank	[tæŋk]
4. thank	[θæŋk]	14. ink	[ɪŋk]
5. rink	[rɪŋk]	15. think	[θɪŋk]
6. link	[lɪŋk]	16. oink	[ɔɪŋk]
7. mink	[mɪŋk]	17. drink	[drɪŋk]
8. blank	[blæŋk]	18. wink	[wɪŋk]
9. cufflink	[kʌflɪŋk]	19. Hank	[hæŋk]
10. dank	[dæŋk]	20. shrink	[ʃrɪŋk]

Exercise 7.22 Identify the following words:

1. /mædi/	Maddie	6. /keli/	Kayle
2. /grɛʧɛn/	Gretchen	7. /ɛli/	Ellie
3. /səmænθə/	Samantha	8. /traɪdɛnt/	trident
4. /dɑLfɪn/	dolphin	9. /paɪntri/	pine tree
5. /gemkɑks/	Gamecocks	10. /krɛsɛnt/	crescent

Exercise 7.24

Down	Across
1. meaning [minɪŋ]	1. men [mɛn]
2. map [mæp]	2. name [næm]
	3. ping [pɪŋ]

Exercise 7.25 Circle the feature(s) that the phonemes have in common:

Manner- Place- Voice

1. /ʃ ŋ/		16. /p n/	
2. /ʧ ʒ/	P	17. /j r/	P V
3. /p n/		18. /r v/	V
4. /m b/	P V	19. /k n/	
5. /s l/		20. /k v/	
6. /ʒ ʤ/	P V	21. /h t/	V
7. /m n/	M V	22. /t f/	V
8. /ʃ t/	V	23. /r ʃ/	P
9. /w j/	M V	24. /l r/	M V
10. /s n/	P	25. /v h/	M
11. /d g/	M	26. /j k/	
12. /m g/	V	27. /f v/	M P
13. /θ ð/	M P	28. /n ʤ/	V
14. /ʃ ʧ/	P V	29. /ʧ j/	P
15. /ʧ ʤ/	M P	30. /g l/	V

Exercise 7.26 Change the listed feature(s) for the onset (phoneme in the initial position) of each word to create a minimal pair. Be sure to use the International Phonetic Alphabet (IPA):

	Manner- Place- Voice	
1. mast	M V	/pæst/ /væst/ /fæst/
2. care	M P	/fɛr/ /tɛr/ /pɛr/ /ʃɛr/ /hɛr/
3. take	P	/kek/
4. pan	M V	/mæn/
5. band	M P	/lænd/
6. date	M P V	/fet/ /het/
7. sell	M	/tɛl/ /pɛl/
8. hen	M P	/pɛn/ /tɛn/ /kɛn/
9. met	M	/bɛt/ /wɛt/
10. chin	M P	/fɪn/pɪn/ /tɪn/ /sɪn/
11. king	M P	/sɪŋ//θɪŋ/
12. kit	P	/pɪt/
13. hoe	M P	/to/
14. might	P	/naɪt/
15. shut	P	/hut/
16. phone	P V	/zon/
17. bite	M P V	/saɪt/
18. rich	M P	/dɪʧ/
19. dutch	M P	/mʌʧ/
20. dam	M V	/sæm/

Exercise 7.27 What is wrong with the following words? If a word is transcribed incorrectly, correctly transcribe it. If a word is transcribed correctly, write "okay":

1. bigger	[bɪgɝ]	[bɪgɚ]
2. shut	[shʌt]	[ʃʌt]
3. bake	[bek]	okay
4. pepper	[pɛppɚ]	[pɛpɚ]
5. bother	[bɑθɚ]	[bɑðɚ]
6. bird	[bɪrd]	[bɝd]
7. black	[blæck]	[blæk]
8. panther	[pænthɚ]	[pænθɚ]
9. sink	[sɪnk]	[sɪŋk]
10. Dutch	[dʌttʃ]	[dʌtʃ]
11. king	[kɪŋ]	okay
12. bomb	[bɑmb]	[bɑm]
13. stow	[stow]	[sto]
14. might	[maɪt]	okay
15. shop	[ʃɑp]	[ʃɑp]
16. phone	[fone]	[fon]
17. bite	[baɪte]	[baɪt]
18. case	[cese]	[kes]
19. supper	[sʌppɚ]	[sʌpɚ]
20. box	[bɑx]	[bɑks]
21. juice	[jus]	[dʒus]

(*Continued*)

22. pegs	[pɛgs]	[pɛgz]
23. wrong	[wrɔŋ]	[rɔŋ]
24. hope	[hope]	[hop]
25. picked	[pɪkɛd]	[pɪkt]

CHAPTER 8

Exercise 8.1 Transcribe the following words showing the heavy aspiration of voiceless stops:

1. key	[kʰi]	6. bane	[ben]
2. game	[gem]	7. touch	[tʰʌʧ]
3. Tom	[tʰɑm]	8. cash	[kʰæʃ]
4. pin	[pʰɪn]	9. pear	[pʰɛr]
5. car	[kʰɑr]	10. dime	[daɪm]

Exercise 8.2 Transcribe the following words showing the release of voiceless stops without heavy aspiration:

1. sicker	[sɪk=ɚ]	6. whisker	[wɪsk=ɚ]
2. spin	[sp=ɪn]	7. detail	[dit=el̩]
3. speak	[sp=ik]	8. stain	[st=en]
4. star	[st=ɑr]	9. scar	[sk=ɑr]
5. sky	[sk=aɪ]	10. checker	[ʧɛk=ɚ]

Exercise 8.3 Transcribe the following words showing unreleased stops:

1. laptop	[læp̚tɑp̚]	6. hope	[hop̚]
2. skateboard	[sket̚bɔrd̚]	7. hog	[hɔg̚]
3. sidecar	[saɪd̚kɑr]	8. fig	[fɪg̚]
4.mitt	[mɪt̚]	9. sideboard	[saɪd̚bɔrd̚]
5. nope	[nop̚]	10. leap	[lip̚]

Exercise 8.4 Transcribe the following words showing the appropriate release and aspiration of all stops:

1. Razorback	[rezɚbæk̚]	6. date	[det̚]
2. pickpocket	[pʰɪk̚pʰɑk=ɛt̚]	7. stick	[st=ɪk̚]
3. steep	[st=ip̚]	8. custard	[kʰʌst=ɚd̚]
4. backpack	[bæk̚pʰæk̚]	9. Gamecock	[gemkʰɑk̚]
5. ductape	[dʌk̚tʰep̚]	10. stop	[st=ɑp̚]

Exercise 8.5 Transcribe the following words showing the influence of nasality on vowels:

1. Tom	[tɑ̃m]	6. pan	[pæ̃n]
2. tone	[tõn]	7. name	[nẽm]
3. tan	[tæ̃n]	8. Ming	[mɪ̃ŋ]
4. meme	[mĩm]	9. can	[kæ̃n]
5. sing	[sɪ̃ŋ]	10. ma'am	[mæ̃m]

Exercise 8.6 Transcribe the following words showing the dentalization of alveolar phonemes:

1. one that	[wən̪ðæt]	6. on this	[ɑn̪ðɪs]
2. synthetic	[sɪn̪θɛtɪk]	7. anthem	[æñ̪θʌm]
3. enthuse	[ɛn̪θuz]	8. ninth	[naɪn̪θ]
4. menthol	[mɛn̪θɔL]	9. Anthony	[æn̪θəni]
5. panther	[pæn̪θɚ]	10. menthol	[mɛn̪θɔL]

Exercise 8.7 Transcribe the following words showing the appropriate lateral allophone:

1. elk	[ɛLk]	6. loathe	[ᶅoð]
2. quell	[kwɛL]	7. Braille	[brɛL]
3. polka	[poLkə]	8. look	[ᶅuk]
4. oil	[ɔɪL]	9. led	[ᶅɛd]
5. late	[ᶅet]	10. eel	[iL]

Exercise 8.8 Transcribe the following words showing the devoicing of liquids in voiceless stop and voiceless fricatives:

1. groom	[grum]	6. sleet	[sl̥it]
2. clue	[kl̥u]	7. plum	[pl̥ʌm]
3. floor	[fl̥ɔr]	8. pride	[pr̥aɪd]
4. slam	[sl̥æm]	9. stream	[strim]
5. blood	[blʌd]	10. tray	[tr̥e]

Exercise 8.9 Transcribe the following words showing lengthening of abutting phonemes:

1. fish shop	[fɪʃ:ɑp]	6. sweet talk	[swit:ɔLk]
2. hot tip	[hɑt:ɪp]	7. homemade	[hom:ed]
3. good day	[gʊd:e]	8. pick corn	[pɪk:ɔrn]
4. nice Sunday	[naɪs:ʌnde]	9. sit tall	[sɪt:ɔL]
5. blood donor	[blʌd:onɚ]	10. this soap	[ðɪs:op]

Exercise 8.10 Transcribe the following words showing use of syllabic consonants:

1. middle	[mɪdL̩]	6. tattle	[tætL̩]
2. bitten	[bɪtn̩]	7. pillar	[pɪlɚ]
3. brittle	[brɪtL̩]	8. mitten	[mɪtn̩]
4. brother	[brɑðɚ]	9. kettle	[kɛtL̩]
5. panel	[pænL̩]	10. dimple	[dɪmpL̩]

Exercise 8.11 Transcribe the following words showing use of glottal stops before syllabic consonants:

1. button	[bʌʔn̩]	6. lighten	[laɪʔn̩]
2. mitten	[mɪʔn̩]	7. fittin'	[fɪʔn̩]
3. Latin	[læʔn̩]	8. mutton	[mʌʔn̩]
4. fatten	[fæʔn̩]	9. satin	[sæʔn̩]
5. batten	[bæʔn̩]	10. written	[rɪʔn̩]

Exercise 8.12 Transcribe the following words showing partial voicing of the intervocalic /t/:

1. metal	[mɛt̬l̩]	6. litter	[lɪt̬ɚ]
2. latter	[læt̬ɚ]	7. pretty	[prɛt̬i]
3. bitter	[bɪt̬ɚ]	8. letter	[lɛt̬ɚ]
4. butter	[bʌt̬ɚ]	9. later	[let̬ɚ]
5. atom	[æt̬m̩]	10. pattern	[pætɚn]

Exercise 8.13 Make the following nouns plural:

1. hog	[hɑgz]	11. wreath	[riθs]
2. girl	[gɝLz]	12. herb	[ɝbz]
3. shoe	[ʃuz]	13. letter	[lɛtɚz]
4. sloth	[slɑθs]	14. judge	[ʤʌʤɛz] or [ʤʌʤɪz]
5. birthmark	[bɝθmɑrks]	15. pattern	[pætɚnz]
6. bush	[bʊʃɛz] or [bʊʃɪz]	16. plate	[plets]
7. chair	[ʧɛrz]	17. pillow	[pɪloz]
8. couch	[koʊʧɛz] or [koʊʧɪz]	18. one	[wʌnz]
9. rug	[rʌgz]	19. tube	[tubz]
10. boat	[bots]	20. clock	[klɑks]

Exercise 8.14 Make the following verbs past tense:

1. smooth	[smuðd]	10. stop	[stɑpt]
2. hop	[hɑpt]	11. include	[ɪnkludɛd] or [ɪnkludɪd]
3.buzz	[bʌzd]	12. need	[nidɛd] or [nidɪd]
4. ask	[æskt]	13. work	[wɝkt]
5. follow	[fɑloz]	14. seem	[simd]
6. alert	[əlɝtɛd] or [əlɝtɪd]	15. camp	[kæmpt]
7. blush	[blʌʃt]	16. cheat	[ʧitɛd] or [ʧitɪd]
8. chew	[ʧud]	17. beg	[bɛgd]
9. brake	[brekt]	18. arrest	[ərɛstɛd] or [ərestɪd]

CHAPTER 9

Exercise 9.1 Transcribe the following words showing the presence of hypernasality:

1. wet	[w̃ɛ̃t]	6. feud	[fj̃ũd]
2. your	[j̃ɔ̃r̃]	7.quit	[kw̃ɪ̃t]
3. weed	[w̃ĩd]	8. we	[w̃ĩ]
4. way	[w̃ẽ]	9. wake	[w̃ẽk]
5. yuck	[j̃ʌ̃k]	10. yard	[j̃ɑ̃r̃d]

Exercise 9.2 Transcribe the following words showing the presence of nasal emission:

1. chick	[ʧ͋ɪk͋]	6. juice	[ʤ͋us͋]
2. pup	[p͋ʌp͋]	7. pot	[pɑt͋]
3. shoe	[ʃ͋u]	8. ship	[ʃ͋ɪp͋]
4. shut	[ʃ͋ʌt͋]	9. zoo	[z͋u]
5. big	[b͋ɪg͋]	10. peach	[p͋iʧ͋]

Exercise 9.3 Transcribe the following words showing the presence of hyponasality:

1. none	[n͊ʌn͊]	6. game	[gem͊]
2. mean	[m͊in͊]	7. matt	[m͊æt]
3. name	[n͊em͊]	8. fun	[fʌn͊]
4. sing	[sɪŋ͊]	9. mutts	[m͊ʌts]
5. birthmark	[bɝθm͊ɑrk]	10. pattern	[pætɚn͊]

Exercise 9.4 Transcribe the following words showing the presence of a frontal lisp:

1. zip	[z̪ɪp]	6. buzz	[bʌz̪]
2. cousin	[kʌz̪ɛn]	7. pencil	[pɛns̪L̩]
3. blossom	[blɑs̪əm]	8. pose	[poz̪]
4. soul	[s̪oL]	9. sank	[s̪æŋk]
5. south	[s̪aʊθ]	10. city	[s̪ɪti]

Exercise 9.5 Transcribe the following words showing the presence of a lateral lisp:

1. seven	[ʪɛvən]	6. stanza	[ʪtænʫə]
2. Samantha	[ʪəmænθə]	7. silly	[ʪɪli]
3. fancy	[fænʪi]	8. graze	[greʫ]
4. satire	[ʪætaɪr]	9. czar	[ʫɑr]
5. hose	[hoʫ]	10. cedar	[ʪidɚ]

Exercise 9.6 Transcribe the following words showing the presence of a palatal /s/:

1. zipper	[zʲɪpɚ]	6. lazy	[lezʲi]
2. sink	[sʲɪŋk]	7. scissors	[sʲɪzʲɚzʲ]
3. sue	[sʲu]	8. zeal	[zʲiL]
4. soap	[sʲop]	9. Xanadu	[zʲænədu]
5. zone	[zʲon]	10. moose	[musʲ]

CHAPTER 10

Exercise 10.1 Transcribe the following words showing weak syllable deletion:

1. tomato	[medo]	6. surprise	[paɪz]
2. spaghetti	[gɛti]	7. refrigerator	[frɪʤretɚ]
3. spider web	[spaɪwɛb]	8. pajamas	[ʤɑməz]
4. dinosaur	[daɪsɔr]	9. helicopter	[hɛlkɑptɚ]
5. vitamin	[vaɪmɪn]	10. watermelon	[wɑmɛlən]

Exercise 10.2 Transcribe the following words showing the effect of final consonant deletion (FCD) or initial consonant deletion (ICD). If one of the following error patterns is not possible, write NP:

Target:	FCD	ICD
1. shoe	NP	[u]
2. Jeff	[ʤɛ]	[ɛf]
3. nope	[no]	[op]
4. though	NP	[o]
5. eat	[i]	NP
6. mash	[mæ]	[æʃ]
7. say	NP	[e]
8. kite	[kaɪ]	[aɪt]
9. cop	[kɑ]	[ɑp]
10. juice	[ʤu]	[us]

Exercise 10.3 Transcribe the following words showing epenthesis:

1. spoon	[səpun]	6. please	[pəliz]
2. spot	[səpɑt]	7. crown	[kəraʊn]
3. black	[bəlæk]	8. stop	[sətɑp]
4. tree	[təri]	9. trapper	[təræpɚ]
5. grape	[gərep]	10. play	[pəle]

Exercise 10.4 Transcribe the following words showing reduplication:

1. cookie	[kʊkʊ]	6. blanket	[bæŋkbæŋk]
2. mitten	[mɪmɪ]	7. television	[tɛLtɛL]
3. supper	[sʌpsʌp]	8. zipper	[zɪpzɪp]
4. napkin	[næpnæp	9. butter	[bʌbʌ]
5. pillow	[pɪLpɪL]	10. middle	[mɪmɪ]

Exercise 10.5 Transcribe the following words showing diminutization:

1. hog	[hɑgi]	6. soap	[sopi]
2. cup	[kʌpi]	7. comb	[komi]
3. doll	[dɔli]	8. bath	[bæθi]
4. coat	[koti]	9. clown	[klaʊni]
5. lamp	[læmpi]	10. juice	[ʤusi]

Exercise 10.6 Transcribe the following words showing cluster reduction or deletion. If cluster reduction or deletion is not possible for the word, write NP:

1. snow	[no]	6. tack	NP
2. skate	[ket]	7. jump	[ʤʌ]
3. star	[tɑr]	8. glue	[gʌ]
4. black	[bæk]	9. wish	NP
5. path	NP	10. beast	[bit]

Exercise 10.7 Transcribe the following words showing stopping.

1. shut	[tʌt]	6. shoe	[tu]
2. juice	[dut]	7. sun	[tʌn]
3. thirsty	[dɝti]	8. ship	[tɪp]
4. soup	[tup]	9. zipper	[dɪpɚ]
5. fish	[pɪt]	10. vase	[bet]

Exercise 10.8 Transcribe the following words showing stridency deletion:

1. hush	[hʌ]	6. cash	[kæt]
2. zoo	[du]	7. Sue	[tu]
3. thief	[θi]	8. finger	[tɪŋgɚ]
4. sugar	[tʊgɚ]	9. vet	[bɛt]
5. pencil	[pɛntʊL]	10. gross	[gro]

Exercise 10.9 Transcribe the following words showing fronting:

1. show	[to]	6. juice	[dus]
2. game	[dem]	7. hog	[hɑd]
3. goat	[dot]	8. kitten	[tɪtn̩]
4. car	[tɑr]	9. cake	[tet]
5. cape	[tep]	10. girl	[dɝL]

Exercise 10.10 Transcribe the following words showing depalatalization:

1. wash	[wɑt]	6. church	[tɝt]
2. shut	[tʌt]	7. judge	[dʌd]
3. juice	[dus]	8. beige	[bed]
4. push	[pt]	9. shoot	[sut]
5. ship	[tɪp]	10. wish	[wɪs]

Exercise 10.11 Transcribe the following words showing alveolarization:

1. pear	[tɛr]	6. thought	[tɑt]
2. bear	[tɛr]	7. thin	[tɪn]
3. thing	[tɪŋ]	8. pig	[tɪg]
4. vase	[des]	9. bat	[tæt]
5. thirsty	[tɝsti]	10. fat	[tæt]

Exercise 10.12 Transcribe the following words showing labialization:

1. tap	[pæp]	6. thick	[pɪk]
2. tore	[pɔr]	7. thigh	[paɪ]
3. door	[pɔr]	8. tan	[pæn]
4. dear	[pɛr]	9. soap	[bop]
5. thank	[pæŋk]	10. sick	[fɪk]

Exercise 10.13 Transcribe the following words showing gliding:

1. lake	[wek]	6. rope	[wop]
2. lady	[jedi]	7. carrot	[kɛwət]
3. rabbit	[wæbɪt]	8. leg	[jɛg]
4. like	[jaɪk]	9. yellow	[jɛjo]
5. rat	[wæt]	10. leap	[wip]

Exercise 10.14 Transcribe the following words showing vowelization:

1. car	[kɑ]	6. sister	[sɪstə]
2. tiger	[taɪgə]	7. mother	[mʌðə]
3. model	[mɑdo]	8. star	[stɑ]
4. little	[lɪto]	9. table	[tebo]
5. burn	[bʌn]	10. bigger	[bɪgə]

Exercise 10.15 Transcribe the following words showing labial assimilation:

1. bat	[bæb]	6. hop	[pɑb]
2. fat	[fæp]	7. home	[mom]
3. boot	[bup]	8. book	[bʊm]
4. mitt	[mip]	9. make	[mem]
5. moat	[mob]	10. pan	[pæp]

Exercise 10.16 Transcribe the following words showing alveolar assimilation:

1. got	[dɑt]	6. dig	[dɪd]
2. tip	[tɪd]	7. hit	[dɪt]
3. Maddie	[dædi]	8. pot	[tɑt]
4. fat	[tæt]	9. top	[tɑt]
5. nope	[not]	10. cheat	[tit]

Exercise 10.17 Transcribe the following words showing velar assimilation:

1. keep	[kik]	6. park	[kɑrk]
2. gate	[geg]	7. hog	[kɑg]
3. goat	[gok]	8. fig	[gɪg]
4. kiss	[kɪk]	9. fork	[kɔrk]
5. pick	[gɪk]	10. Kim	[kɪg]

Exercise 10.18 Transcribe the following words showing nasal assimilation:

1. map	[mæn]	6. phone	[mon]
2. pink	[nɪŋk]	7. fame	[mem]
3. Pam	[mæm]	8. mate	[mæn]
4. tone	[non]	9. note	[non]
5. nope	[non]	10. more	[mon]

Exercise 10.19 Transcribe the following words showing prevocalic voicing:

1. take	[dek]	6. tiger	[daɪgɚ]
2. pan	[bæn]	7. cow	[daʊ]
3. soap	[dop]	8. pain	[ben]
4. ship	[ʤɪp]	9. chair	[ʤɛr]
5. sit	[zɪt]	10. cake	[gek]

Exercise 10.20 Transcribe the following words showing postvocalic devoicing:

1. rag	[ræk]	6. Hogue	[hop]
2. skid	[skɪt]	7. hog	[hɔk]
3. side	[saɪt]	8. maze	[mes]
4. pad	[pæt]	9. jab	[ʤæp]
5. knob	[nɑp]	10. made	[met]

FLASH CARDS

/k/	/g/	/p/
/b/	/t/	/d/
/s/	/z/	/f/

#1 Voiceless Lingua-Velar Stop-Consonant /k/ Initial cat /**k**æb/ Medial across /ʌ**k**rɔs/ Final bake /be**k**/	#4 Voiced Bilabial Stop-Consonant /b/ Initial bat /**b**æt/ Medial above /ʌ**b**əv/ Final lab /læ**b**/	#7 Voiceless Lingua-Alveolar Fricative /s/ Initial sat /**s**æt/ Medial listen /lɪ**s**ɛn/ Final hiss /hɪ**s**/
#2 Voiced Lingua-Velar Stop-Consonant /g/ Initial game /**g**em/ Medial regret /ri**g**rɛt/ Final log /la**g**/	#5 Voiceless Lingua-Alveolar Stop-Consonant /t/ Initial take /**t**ek/ Medial atop /ʌ**t**ap/ Final spot /spa**t**/	#8 Voiced Lingua Alveolar Fricatived /z/ Initial zoo /**z**u/ Medial ozone /o**z**on/ Final blaze /ble**z**/
#3 Voiceless Bilabial Stop-Consonant /p/ Initial pitch /**p**ɪʧ/ Medial open /o**p**ɛn/ Final cape /ke**p**/	#6 Voiced Lingua-Alveolar Stop-Consonant /d/ Initial dog /**d**ag/ Medial ladder /læ**d**ɚ/ Final card /kar**d**/	#9 Voiceless Labiodental Fricative /f/ Initial fig /**f**ɪg/ Medial stuffy /stʌ**f**i/ Final staff /stæ**f**/

/ʧ/	/ʃ/	/v/
/ʤ/	/ʒ/	/θ/
/hw/	/h/	/ð/

#10
Voiced Labiodental Fricative /v/

Initial	vote	/vot/
Medial	clover	/klovɚ/
Final	love	/lʌv/

#13
Voiceless Lingua-Palatal Fricative /ʃ/

Initial	shake	/ʃek/
Medial	mushroom	/mʌʃrum/
Final	push	/puʃ/

#16
Voiceless Alveopalatal Affricate /ʧ/

Initial	change	/ʧeŋʤ/
Medial	teacher	/tiʧɚ/
Final	peach	/piʧ/

#11
Voiceless Interdental Fricative /θ/

Initial	thank	/θaŋk/
Medial	bathroom	/baθrum/
Final	path	/pæθ/

#14
Voiced Lingua-Palatal Fricative /ʒ/

Initial	Does not exist	
Medial	leisure	/liʒɚ/
Final	beige	/beʒ/

#17
Voiced Alveopalatal Affricate /ʤ/

Initial	gem	/ʤɛm/
Medial	gadget	/gæʤɛt/
Final	fudge	/fʌʤ/

#12
Voiced Interdental Fricative /ð/

Initial	this	/ðɪs/
Medial	mother	/mʌðɚ/
Final	bathe	/beð/

#15
Voiceless Glottal Fricative /h/

Initial	help	/hɛlp/
Medial	ahead	/ʌhɛd/
Final	Does not exist in	

#18
Voiceless Labial-Velar Fricative /hw/

Initial	when	/hwɛn/
Medial	bushwhack	/buʃhwæk/
Final	Does not exist	

/m/	/n/	/ŋ/
/l/	/j/	/r/
/w/	/i/	/ɪ/

#19 Voiced Bilabial Nasal /m/ Initial mode /**m**od/ Medial amazing /ʌ**m**azɪŋ/ Final dam /dæ**m**/	#22 Voiced Lingua-Alveolar Lateral Liquid /l/ Initial lift /**l**ɪft/ Medial jolly /ʤa**l**i/ Final doll /da**l**/	#25 Voiced Bilabial Glide /w/ Initial wet /**w**ɛt/ Medial jomework /hom**w**ɚk/ Final Does not exist
#20 Voiced Lingua-Alveolar Nasal /n/ Initial name /**n**em/ Medial control /kʌ**n**trol/ Final man /mæ**n**/	#23 Voiced Lingua-Palatal On-Glide /j/ Initial yak /**j**æk/ Medial reuse /ri**j**us/ Final Does not exist	#26 High Front Unrounded Vowel /i/ Initial eat /**i**t/ Medial street /str**i**t/ Final fee /f**i**/
#21 Voiced Velar Nasal /ŋ/ Initial Does not exist Medial anger /e**ŋ**gɚ/ Final bring /brɪ**ŋ**/	#24 Voiced Alveo-Palatal Liquid /r/ Initial rock /**r**ak/ Medial rubric /rub**r**ɪk/ Final star /sta**r**/	#27 Mid-High Front Unrounded Vowel /ɪ/ Initial instant /**ɪ**nstænt/ Medial spin /sp**ɪ**n/ Final gritty /grɪt**ɪ**/

/ɑ/	/u/	/e/
/ɔ/	/ʊ/	/ɛ/
	/o/	/æ/

#28
Mid Front Unrounded Vowel /e/

Initial	ape	/**e**p/
Medial	staple	/st**e**pl/
Final	stray	/str**e**/

#29
Mid-Low Front Unrounded Vowel /ɛ/

Initial	egg	/**e**g/
Medial	get	/gɛt/
Final	Does not exist	

#30
Low Front Unrounded Vowel /æ/

Initial	at	/**æ**t/
Medial	that	/ð**æ**t/
Final	Does not exist	

#31
High Back Rounded Vowel /u/

Initial	shoe	/ʃ**u**/
Medial	dual	/d**u**l/
Final	flu	/fl**u**/

#32
Mid-High Back Rounded Vowel /ʊ/

Initial	Does not exist	
Medial	book	/b**ʊ**k/
Final	Does not exist	

#33
Mid Back Rounded Vowel /o/

Initial	open	/**o**pɛn/
Medial	stone	/st**o**n/
Final	hello	/hɛl**o**/

#34
Mid-Low Back Rounded Vowel /ɔ/

Initial	awesome	/**ɔ**səm/
Medial	brawl	/br**ɔ**l/
Final	straw	/str**ɔ**/

#35
Low Back Rounded Vowel /ɑ/

Initial	olive	/**ɑ**lɪv/
Medial	hot	/h**ɑ**t/
Final	sofa	/sof**ɑ**/

/ɝ/	/j͜u/	/ɔ͜ɪ/
/ɚ/	/ʌ/	/a͜ʊ/
	/ə/	/a͜ɪ/

#37 Mid-Low Back Rounded to High Front Unrounded Diphthong /ɔ͜ɪ/ Initial oyster /ɔ͜ɪstɚ/ Medial royal /rɔ͜ɪl/ Final joy /ʤɔ͜ɪ/	#40 Lingua-Palatal On-Glide to High Back Rounded Diphthong /j͜u/ Initial you /j͜u/ Medial feud /fj͜ud/ Final few /fj͜u/	#43 Mid-High Closed Middle Vowel /ɝ/ Initial Earth /ɝθ/ Medial bird /bɝd/ Final Does not exist
#38 Low Back Rounded to Mid-High Back Rounded Diphthong /a͜ʊ/ Initial ouch /a͜ʊʧ/ Medial cowbell /ka͜ʊbɛl/ Final bow /ba͜ʊ/	#41 Mid-Low Closed Middle Vowel /ʌ/ Initial up /ʌp/ Medial above /əbʌv/ Final Does not exist	#44 Mid Closed Middle Vowel /ɚ/ Initial Does not exist Medial Does not exist Final father /fɑðɚ/
#39 Low Back Rounded to Mid-High Front Unrounded Diphthong /a͜ɪ/ Initial ice /a͜ɪs/ Medial twice /twa͜ɪs/ Final tie /ta͜ɪ/	#42 Mid-High Closed Middle Vowel /ə/ Initial above /əbʌv// Medial Does not exist Final Does not exist	

/fʊt/

/mud/

/gedʒ/

/ðɪs/

/ʃek/

/ðiz/

/θɔt/

/hʊk/

/dʒɛt/

/kat/

/ʃʊk/

/bu/

/ʃat/

/no/

/θɔt/

/dʒu/

/liʒɝ/

Stops

/t/
/d/ > CP

/k/
/g/ > CP

/p/
/b/ > CP

Front vowels

/i/ eat
/I/ chicken
/e/ late
/ɛ/ get
/æ/ fat

Back vowels

/u/ New
/ʊ/ Book
/o/ Show
/ɔ/ always
/a/ hot

Affricates

/tʃ/ chip /tʃIp/
/dʒ/ juice /dʒus/

Fricatives

/f/
/v/ > CP

/θ/ Thorn
/ð/ > CP these

/s/ so
/z/ > CP zoo

/ʃ/ ship
/ʒ/ > CP leisure

/h/

CPSIA information can be obtained
at www.ICGtesting.com
Printed in the USA
LVOW02s0047060917
547691LV00005B/21/P